HELP YOUR DOG
FIGHT
CANCER

AN OVERVIEW OF
HOME CARE OPTIONS

FEATURING BULLET'S SURVIVAL STORY

LAURIE KAPLAN

The information in this book applies only to canines. Some therapies, treatments and methods discussed in Help Your Dog Fight Cancer may be harmful if applied to felines or other species of animals with or without cancer.

Please forgive the assignment of masculine pronouns to both humans and canines in this book when they are discussed in general terms. This does not reflect any desire by the author to express sexism, but rather a desire to present the content in the most easily readable format.

Great care has been taken to ensure the accuracy of the information presented in good conscience herein and to ensure that no methods are described that could be harmful to your dog. The author, editor and publisher are not responsible for errors or omissions or for any consequences from the application of the information in this book and make no warranty, express or implied, with regard to the contents of the book. Current procedures, methods and practices are dynamic and subject to change. Although the author, editor and publisher have done everything reasonably possible to make this book accurate and up-to-date, as new scientific information becomes available through basic and clinical research and studies, recommended treatments and procedures undergo changes. The advice and strategies contained herein may not be suitable for your situation. Individual canine anatomy, physiology, requirements and capabilities vary and specific recommendations applicable may not be appropriate for a particular dog. This book is not intended as veterinary medical advice nor to supplant appropriate veterinary medical consultation. Readers are advised to always consult with a veterinarian regarding these matters.

Library of Congress Control Number: 2004107152
ISBN: 0-9754794-6-6

Cover photograph by Tracy M. Basile
Cover design by Kim Leonard/Bookcovers.com
Publishing coach: Allen D'Angelo MS, Archer-Ellison, Inc.

CONTENTS

SPECIAL INFORMATION

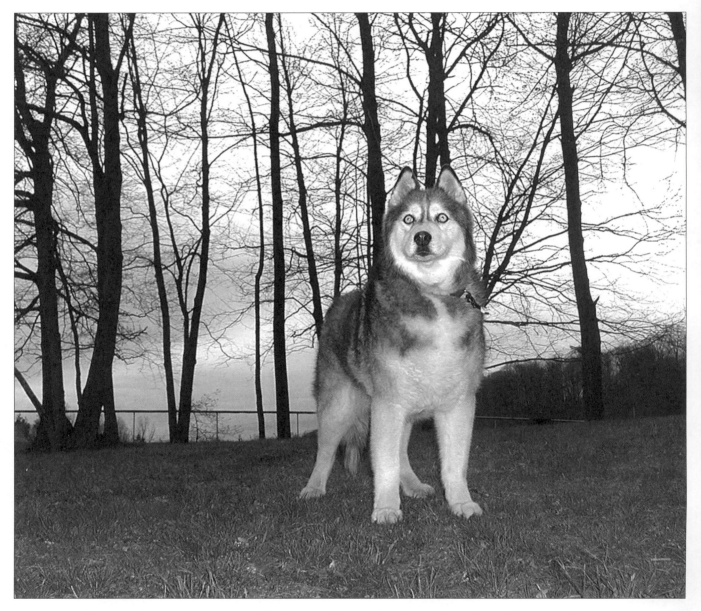

Dedicated to my brave little boy The love of my life The dog of my dreams The Magic Bullet

Author's Preface

Experts predict that approximately half of our dogs will have cancer in their lifetimes and yet, as caretakers, most of us know little or nothing about caring for a dog with cancer. Not long ago, admittedly, there wasn't much to know. Today, however, treatment for canine cancer is nearly on a par with treatment for human cancer and there is a great deal to know.

If your dog has cancer, you're undoubtedly asking, "What can I do?" First, you'll see that a medical plan is decided upon and put into action. This book will help you to decide on a plan and to decide how active a role you will play in your dog's fight against cancer. You'll read about the treatment options for canine cancer and the types of decisions that you can be involved in making right from the start. Whatever degree of involvement you choose, *Help Your Dog Fight Cancer* will help you on your way.

Once a medical plan has been decided upon, you'll ask, "What else can I do?" Lots! Regardless of what type of medical treatment you choose (chemotherapy, radiation, surgery, an alternative therapy or no treatment at all), there is a great deal more that you can do. You'll learn how to manage symptoms and side effects, strengthen your dog's organs and bolster his system. You'll learn how to help your dog better fight the disease and better tolerate the treatment and perhaps you'll improve his odds for survival.

When Bullet was diagnosed with cancer, I wanted to know what could, might and typically does happen in such cases. I wanted to know what I should, shouldn't, could and might do to help him survive. Moreover, I wanted to know all of this right away and in plain English.

I was disheartened, finding no book that would help me understand the typical course of events, the options, the possible pitfalls, how to deal with them and what to expect—best case and worst. I set about learning all I could as quickly as I could, as many devoted and terrified cancer-dog caretakers have done in recent years. My experience as an animal writer and editor of medical literature hadn't educated me about canine cancer in any way that would be helpful to me as the caretaker of a cancer-dog, but did enable me to wade through medical literature reasonably undaunted by medical lingo and to write this book.

During the first year of Bullet's cancer treatment, I consulted general practice veterinarians, veterinary oncologists, holistic vets, oncologists in human medicine and other caretakers of dogs with cancer. I read books both medical and lay to research medications, supplements, nutraceuticals, diets and clinical trials. I experimented extensively to find the regimen that would work best for both Bullet and me.

The more information I gathered and the more I understood about Bullet's condition, the more capable I felt of caring for him properly and the more my anxiety level diminished. What research didn't teach me, experience did.

Paolo Porzio, DVM, who administered Bullet's chemotherapy, urged me repeatedly to write a book that would help other caretakers of dogs with cancer allay those feelings of anxiety that come from not knowing—the very book that I had not been able to find. After a year of shrugging off Dr. Porzio's urgings, I finally resigned my position as editor-in-chief of *Catnip* magazine, a publication of Tufts University School of Veterinary Medicine, and set about writing this book.

For Bullet's sake, I researched and fact-checked while choosing options for his care. For your dog's sake, I did more research and fact checking while composing this book. Wherever possible, I provide the source of my data. Much of it, however, has been accumulated from undocumented sources or is based on my own experience.

The three key members of Bullet's team—his general practice veterinarian, the doctor who provided chemotherapy and the veterinary oncologist who served as our consultant—have all been kind enough to fact-check the manuscript of *Help Your Dog Fight Cancer* for medical accuracy and to ensure that, according to what is now known about canine cancer, no recommendations are made that might harm a cancer-dog.

Several top-notch veterinarians and veterinary oncologists have each generously contributed to *Help Your Dog Fight Cancer* information in their area of expertise or special interest. No one of these experts endorses every facet of Bullet's home-care program or every recommendation presented in this book.

As you develop a home-care regimen for your dog, discuss your plans with your veterinarian. Include any facets of Bullet's home-care program that you wish to use. Some methods that have worked well for Bullet could be contraindicated for your dog's breed or condition, the type of cancer that he has, his individual sensitivities or the medical treatment he's receiving.

I've helped many caretakers begin the bitter-sweet journey involved in living with and caring for a cancer-dog. All are initially overwhelmed, as I was, by the endless list of decisions to be made. *Help Your Dog Fight Cancer* doesn't contain an encyclopedic listing of treatments, supplements, dosages and diets. Rather, it presents the "short list" for each and shares the shorter list that defines the choices I've made over the years in building a home-care program for my cancer-dog.

There are a thousand ways to care for a dog with cancer and each caretaker has to choose his or her options. I offer no evidence that the care package I've designed for Bullet is responsible for his survival. Without chemotherapy, Bullet would certainly have had no chance of survival longer than the typical one-month prognosticated for dogs with untreated lymphoma. Perhaps Bullet's survival so far beyond his prognosis is due to his hardy constitution and his stubborn personality.

My hope is that every reader will come away from *Help Your Dog Fight Cancer* with a plan and with confidence, prepared to begin the journey. Be creative, flexible, adventurous and careful in caring for your cancer-dog. And keep the faith!

In caring for my cancer-dog and in composing this book, I've taken great pains to discover those treatments and therapies that I believe to have the greatest potential for success from a variety of sources within traditional and holistic medicine.

Cancer is a fierce enemy and to "fight the good fight," we need all the ammunition we can get. *Help Your Dog Fight Cancer* will provide you with a solid foundation for your battle against canine cancer. Armed with information and love, you will discover the best possible way to care for your own cancer-dog.

WITH GRATITUDE

I've been lucky enough to have various types of support from some special people in and around the creation of *Help Your Dog Fight Cancer,* beginning with a top-notch medical team. The excellent care that Bullet received before, during and since the diagnosis of lymphoma was the foundation for his survival and hence for this book.

Bullet's primary-care medical team, including Dr. Bruce Hoskins and the Croton Animal Hospital staff, has kept him healthy and strong for 13 years (and counting).

The expertise of Bullet's cancer team is self-evident in light of his long survival. Dr. Paolo Porzio treated Bullet expertly and lovingly and envisioned *Help Your Dog Fight Cancer* long before I embraced that vision.

Dr. David Ruslander provided guidance in all cancer-related matters during Bullet's cancer treatment and more recently toward the medical accuracy of this book. Amazingly, two baby Ruslanders were brought into the world during the gestation of this one small book.

Doctors Tina Aiken and Marty Goldstein at the Smith Ridge Veterinary Center expanded on Bullet's cancer treatment plan to include a holistic dimension. All of the holistic and alternative components of our home-care program evolved from their initial recommendations.

I'm especially grateful to veterinary oncologists Phil Bergman, Kevin Hahn and Rodney Page who contributed in a very direct fashion. Each composed a page of the book on a topic of their choosing, with an informative and heartfelt message to the reader.

Help Your Dog Fight Cancer would be conspicuously lacking were it not for the contributions of two special veterinarians. Dr. Allen Schoen speaks to readers of the powerful spiritual bond that develops between caretaker and dog during difficult times and Dr. W. Jean Dodds shares her extensive knowledge about the relationship between vaccines and canine cancer.

On a personal note, Bullet's "Aunts and Uncles" have provided emotional support to me and hands-on care for Bullet. Thank you, Kevin Griffin, Catriona Lappell, Andrea Rabe, Tracy Basile, Connie Schwarting, Tom Sweeney, Alice Shanahan and Martha Kenerson, Rick and Abby Kaplan.

Finally, I thank the Perseus Foundation, a non-profit organization that boasts a unique board of directors including veterinary oncologists and human oncologists working side by side with the common goal of treating, researching and curing cancer.

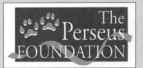

In honor of Bullet and concurrent with the publication of this book, the Perseus Foundation will announce the inception of THE MAGIC BULLET FUND. This new fund provides low-cost canine cancer treatment for selected cancer-dogs from coast to coast when caretakers cannot bear the financial burden.

The creation of this fund is possible due to donations from corporate sponsors. The day-to-day work and operating costs of the fund are dependent on donations from dog lovers who believe that every cancer-dog deserves a chance to survive cancer. Please see page 109 for more information about The Magic Bullet Fund.

THE MAGIC BULLET

~ PART ONE

I must take this opportunity to tell Bullet's story and to claim for him the "15 minutes of fame" that is most certainly his due. If your dog has been diagnosed with cancer and you are feeling overwhelmed, please skip "Bullet's Story" and go directly to Chapter 1.

'd lived with cats for many years—15 cats in all, but never more than three at a time for fear of earning the title "the cat lady." On September 19, 1992, I was toying with the idea of sharing my home with a dog in addition to my three resident felines, KC, Bumi and TipToe. I wandered into the local animal shelter from which I had adopted TipToe a year earlier, intending only to hand out biscuits to the pups and explore my feelings about bringing a new member, of the canine species, into the family.

My friend Kevin and I perused the canine residents, handed out biscuits to many and took a few for walks in the shelter parking lot. Then, Kevin pointed out a dog in one of the large outdoor cages. The ID tag hanging on the cage indicated that this was Max, an 18-month-old neutered male Siberian Husky. Max was sitting quietly amidst the chaos generated by several other medium-to-large dogs who cohabited the cage, all barking wildly and vying for position to receive biscuits.

Max had the most beautiful ears and eyes I'd ever seen. He was strikingly black and white with a handsome star-shaped design on his chest. I looked at Max and he looked at me. It was a bit unnerving, being studied with such intensity by two icy blue eyes in a canine head. Love at first sight? Maybe so—in any case, I knew then and there that this dog with super-canine eye contact was going to be mine.

According to the shelter manager, the Husky had been relinquished by his owner the previous day. The owner complained that Max was an escape artist and a "runner." Apparently, he had bailed Max out, for a fee, one time too many.

I've since learned, by reading up on the breed and by chasing Bullet down many, many times, that it's redundant to say a dog is a Siberian Husky *and* a runner. In fact, I had an opportunity to witness the Siberian penchant for escape early on. I had Max taken from his kennel and walked him around the parking lot. I then left Kevin holding the leash and I went into the office to pay the suggested $40 donation. When I came out a few minutes later, I found Kevin still holding the leash...only now the leash was dangling to the ground with no dog attached to it. "Oh," Kevin said when he noticed my expression. "You're *taking* that dog?"

A shelter worker and I chased Max down. He seemed to be having great fun watching the three of us over his shoulder and eluding our attempts at capture. Finally, exasperated, I stopped running, clapped my hands and yelled *"MAAAAX!"* To everyone's amazement, Max ran to me from behind a nearby house and rolled over on his back at my feet—an event that would never ever happen again.

Soon thereafter, "Max" became "Bullet" (as in faster than a speeding...) because of his great love of running. His friends call him "Bully" because of his great love of growling.

In our first six months together, Bullet was ousted from three boarding kennels and two professional dog trainers deemed him untrainable. One went so far as to recommend that I return him to the shelter...alas, it was too late. I suspect it was too late from the moment that I put him into my car at the shelter.

In the early years, Bullet destroyed everything in the house that was not nailed down, and a few things that were. He loved nothing more than to chew on (although never bite) a human hand or arm. Periodically, I went in another room and closed the door to give myself a "time out" from Bullet. I was simply exhausted from yelling "NO!" over and over. I came across the movie, *Turner and Hooch* shortly after I adopted Bullet and howled with laughter—I related completely to Turner's (played by Tom Hanks) frustration and exasperation.

As a strong healthy youth, Bullet was a big-time puller "on leash." If only I had a nickel for every time a passer-by said *"Who's walking whom?"* I didn't weigh much more than Bullet and he was capable of pulling me right off my feet, especially if a squirrel, rabbit or cat happened by to provide incentive.

When Bullet encountered unfamiliar dogs, he always became extremely agitated and I was never entirely sure whether he intended to play or fight. I would drag him off-trail, grab onto a tree and hang on until the dog passed by.

In 2001, a friend visited an American Indian Reservation and was inspired to assign new names to our dogs. Her dogs, Kai (lion-hearted deer-dog, friend of the coyotes) and Toshi (frog-dancer, water-prancer) were Bullet's best furry friends for many years. We ceremoniously and quite appropriately dubbed my ornery little boy, "Bullet Growly Bear."

True to the breed, Bullet ran away whenever possible. He could chew through a nylon or leather leash so quickly and surreptitiously that he would be on the run with a healthy head start by the time I realized that he wasn't at the end of the leash. He even managed to get away from one

of the dog trainers who worked with him. Perhaps coincidentally, it was the same trainer who had suggested that I return Bullet to the shelter.

I knew there was nothing wrong with this dog that a lot of tender love (and a lot of *tough* love) couldn't fix. I read dog-training books and books about the Husky personality. What I needed was a how-to book for training a Siberian Husky.

After a few months, a few books and a few new wrinkles on my brow, Bullet became a bit more manageable. After a few years of training (what one friend calls "Laurie's Boot Camp"), Bullet and I finally found a place of mutual respect with me as the Alpha.

Bullet was a ridiculously high maintenance dog. In time, he became a very opinionated but manageable dog. I find that the older he gets, the better he gets and now that he is "geriatric dog," he's nearly perfect.

In his own good time, Bullet did master basic obedience commands such as Sit, Down, Stay, Paw, Other Paw, Jump, Speak and Kiss (this last has always been our favorite), but he never, to this day, learned to "Come" off lead. I'm quite sure it's an auditory problem—Bullet's hearing is just fine with a leash attached, but he reliably goes stone-cold deaf the moment the leash is clicked off from the collar. From my readings and from talking to other frustrated and bemused Siberian caretakers, I gather this hearing problem is genetic.

BULLY'S WORLD

At first, Bullet slept in a finished basement at night. I had planned to introduce him to the cats gradually before allowing him free run of the house. I would go downstairs each morning to find the floor littered with remnants of books, notepads, computer disks, pencils and anything else within his reach. A friend convinced me that Bullet, being a Northern-breed dog, should sleep outdoors. In light of the wreckage, this sounded to me like a great idea.

Bullet moved to the great outdoors, his collar hooked onto an overhead run between two trees, 50 feet apart. He had a doghouse full of hay but chose to sleep under the stars on a second pile of hay except in the most inclement weather. In thunderstorms, he always slept indoors in his room in the basement, even though he had a cozy house for shelter. I had read that outdoor dogs are often struck by lightening.

During the winter, a dog living outdoors can tear his tongue on ice. I had an electrical outlet installed next to the doghouse and purchased a heated water bowl. To make further use of the outlet, I plugged in a baby monitor and placed it in the doghouse. Its counterpart hung beside my bed. More often than I care to remember, I was awakened in the wee hours by frantic barking coming from my end of the baby monitor. De-skunking baths in the front yard at 2 a.m. became commonplace, always followed by a car ride in search of a dumpster while holding a multi-wrapped skunk carcass out of the window as far as possible from my nose.

In 1995, I arranged for a 5-foot high chain-link fence to be installed in the woods behind my house. The resulting dog pen measured 50 feet by 50 feet—larger than the footprint of my house. Furnished with a doghouse, lounge chair and flat-roofed eating station, this pen gave Bullet freedom from the overhead run, put a stop to the skunk carnage and became "Bully's World."

BULLET'S TEACHINGS

Bullet taught me how to train an untrainable dog. He taught me to understand dog-speak and to communicate with him in a way that he could understand. But he taught me much more than this. For example, Bullet inspired me to learn to knit so that I could make sweaters, vests and scarves from his fur.

The fur (undercoat) of any Northern breed dog or any dog that has a double coat can be spun and knitted. Because a dog's fur lacks the elasticity found in strands of a sheep's wool, most spinners blend some amount (10 to 30 percent) of sheep's wool with the dog fur.

Dog fur becomes quite fuzzy when knitted, looking very much like mohair, and the final product is so warm that I was unable to wear my Bully-sweaters indoors. So, I turned sweaters into vests by removing the sleeves. So as not to waste any precious fur, I simply turned the sleeves into slipper-socks.

Bullet also taught me to mush. On winter weekends, we went on dog sledding trips in Lake Placid, NY, where he added a few new commands to his repertoire. These were Hike (start running), Gee (turn right), Haw (turn left), Straight On and Whoa. I rented a cabin on these weekends and rented a sled and three huskies from the owner of a professional Siberian dog sledding team. What a rush! Seeing Bullet take to sledding like a duck to water gave me a new sense of respect for who he is and for the natural order of things.

In 1998, when Bullet was 7, he had surgery on both shoulders to remove a bone chip and debris from the joints. This marked the end of Bullet's sledding days and squashed any fantasies I might have had of running in the Iditarod. The recovery from this surgery was difficult for Bullet. For the first time, it seemed as though this unruly, rebellious and fiercely independent dog was dependent. Unfortunately, before very long, I would be seeing this side of Bullet all too clearly.

THE DISCOVERY OF CANCER

In May 2000, I felt enlarged glands in Bullet's neck, just where a doctor will feel your neck if you complain of a sore throat. Initially, allergy was suspected and antihistamines were prescribed. The enlarged glands remained in spite of the medications and so we paid our veterinarian a visit.

Bullet's lifelong primary care veterinarian, Bruce Hoskins DVM, at Croton Animal Hospital in Croton-on-Hudson, NY, attempted a needle biopsy of a lymph node in order to rule out lymphoma. The fluid extracted did not contain lymph and so a surgical biopsy was performed the following day.

Dr. Hoskins reported that he had taken the biopsy sample from the popliteal lymph node behind Bullet's left knee. The node had all but disintegrated during the procedure, he said, and had to be excised entirely. Still, he was hopeful that if lymphoma was found, it would be an early stage cancer.

The next evening, on July 17, 2000, Dr. Hoskins called to say, "The laboratory report on Bullet's biopsy was positive for lymphoma." I knew that this could not be true. *There must be a mistake.* Aside from the swollen glands I'd found in his neck, Bullet was a strong, healthy 9-year-old Siberian Husky. Physically and behaviorally, he emitted an air of strength, health and heartiness and seemed impervious to illness and injury. Surely, the laboratory got their blood samples mixed up or had misinterpreted the results. "No," I was assured, "there is no mistake."

I was dumfounded. I was shocked. I had a lump in my throat and a knot in my stomach. I stayed up all night, intermittently hugging him, crying, researching canine lymphoma online and contacting anyone and everyone I knew in the field of veterinary medicine or cancer research for advice. I was at that time editor-in-chief of *Catnip* Magazine, a publication from Tufts University School of Veterinary Medicine. The show of support from the top-notch Tufts veterinarians when they learned of Bullet's illness touched, impressed and strengthened me.

STARTING TREATMENT

Dr. Hoskins provided me with the names and telephone numbers of local veterinary oncologists and of a local veterinarian who was not board certified in oncology but provided cancer treatment to dogs and cats. Paolo Porzio, DVM, diplomate ACVIM (internal medicine) is now at the Glen Erin Animal Hospital in Mississauga, Ontario, Canada. But in July 2000, luckily for us, he was at the Tuckahoe Animal Hospital in Tuckahoe, NY, just half an hour away.

Dr. Porzio agreed to start Bullet on chemotherapy the very next day. At first, I chose him to begin Bullet's treatment based on location and availability despite the fact that he was not board certified in oncology. The most important thing, in my mind, was to get Bullet into treatment as quickly as possible.

During our very first visit, however, I knew that Dr. Porzio had been a great choice. He was very attentive to Bullet during our conversation and spoke to him in a sweet, gentle and affectionate way. His "bedside manner" was perfect. He spoke clearly, explained everything to me in an unrushed manner and he took his time answering all of my many questions thoroughly.

Another advantage was that the veterinary office was on the ground floor and the storefront was a huge plate-glass window. This meant that I could see if there were any dogs in the waiting room before entering—a big plus, since Bullet doesn't always take kindly to new dogs. I was relieved to know that there would never be a ruckus in the waiting room or a struggle to keep Bullet from lunging at another dog.

Dr. Porzio completed a residency in veterinary internal medicine in Saskatchewan. Because there was no staff oncologist at the school while Dr. Porzio was enrolled, he and the other interns learned to provide cancer treatment to the dogs. The locale of the doctor's training appealed to me because it meant that Dr. Porzio would have to be familiar with the idiosyncrasies and antics of the breed (and there are many). I've found that not all doctors are enamored by the exuberance and obstinacy of the Siberian Husky.

Dr. Porzio treated many cancer-dogs and his treatment of choice was single-agent (one drug) chemotherapy, with an agent called adriamycin. I consulted several veterinary oncologists, most notably Dave Ruslander, DVM, diplomate ACVIM (Oncology), diplomate ACVR (Radiation Oncology), at the Veterinary Specialty Hospital of the Carolinas in Cary, NC. Dr. Ruslander recommended a treatment plan called VELCAP-L for Bullet's chemotherapy. It was more complex but also showed a higher success rate than the single-agent adriamycin plan. Dr. Porzio readily agreed to use the VELCAP-L treatment plan for Bullet with Dr. Ruslander's guidance. Dr. Ruslander has contributed immeasurably to Bullet's well-being and survival over the years.

Now that I had a medical treatment plan in place, I wanted to know, *"What else can I do?"* The first thing that I did was make an appointment with Marty Goldstein, DVM, renowned holistic veterinarian and author of *The Nature of Animal Healing: The Definitive Holistic Medicine Guide to Caring for Your Dog and Cat*. Dr. Goldstein lifted my spirits and gave me hope. He spoke of many cancer-dogs who had triumphed over cancer and showed me photographs of them. This was my first lesson in supplements for canine cancer.

Bullet's Story continues on page 103.

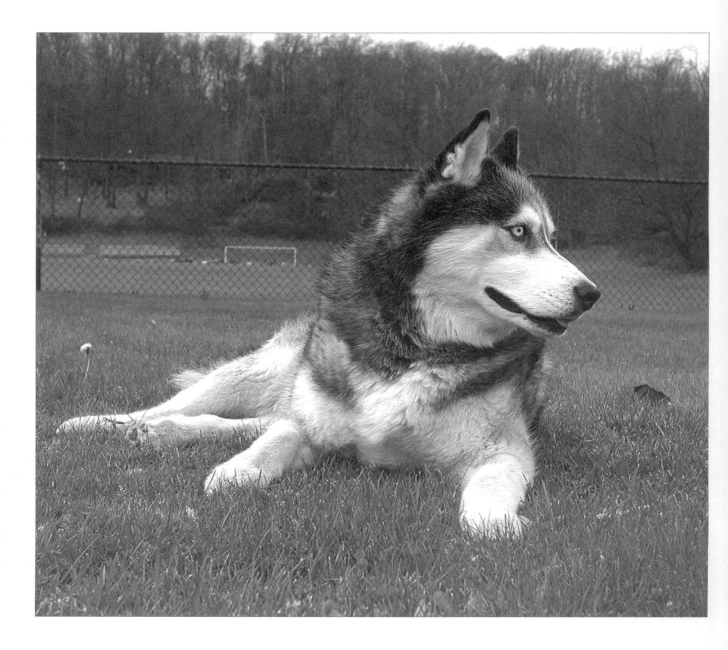

1

PREPARE FOR BATTLE

"Your dog has cancer." Suddenly, your pal, your playful companion, hiking buddy, confidante and protector (or protectee) has become a cancer patient. You no longer look at him with eyes full of happiness and love. Your eyes, your tone of voice, your posture and your energy level all speak of sadness, pity and anger.

Dogs are sensitive to the type of energy (vibes) that their humans send out—our "auras," if you will. Don't let your long face be a "downer" for your dog when he's ill, and especially not when he's feeling well and happy. My message is not to *put on* a happy face, but rather to actually *have* a happy face and a happy heart. Hold him close and let his fur absorb your tears on occasion but, for the main, stay upbeat and positive and be truly grateful and full of joy for the time that he has been with you and because he is with you now. Thoroughly relish every day that you have together and keep reminding yourself that your pal is now on borrowed time and each day is a precious gift.

"How can I pretend to be happy when I'm so sad?" Don't pretend! Tend to your dog. Make him comfortable in any way you can think of and focus your attention on working to pull him through. Use your imagination—even the smallest contributions that you make to improve his comfort level are important.

When you've done everything you can and there's nothing more to do, simply sit by his side, pet him, sing him a song! Bullet has proved to me that dogs like being sung to even if the singer can't carry a tune. If singing is out of the question, then talk to your dog. The sound of your voice will soothe him. Remember to say his name often.

When Bullet was diagnosed with lymphoma, I learned that without chemotherapy, dogs with this disease generally perish within a month. David Ruslander, DVM, diplomate ACVIM (Oncology), diplomate ACVR (Radiation Oncology), at the Veterinary Specialty Hospital of the Carolinas in Cary, NC, informed me that with chemotherapy, 50 percent of dogs with lymphoma survive one year and 25 percent survive two years or more. Many dogs survive various types of cancer for long periods of time. Some enjoy a normal life span and live on to die years later from a completely unrelated cause.

I was afraid to hope that Bullet might be lucky enough to fall into this minority. I liked the sound of a one-year remission, though, because Bullet was just past his ninth birthday when he was diagnosed. A one-year reprieve would afford him a normal life span for a Siberian Husky.

In July of 2000, Bullet had his first visit with Paolo Porzio, DVM, diplomate ACVIM (internal medicine). Dr. Porzio said that he thought Bullet would be very happy when the weather turned cold. I asked (dubiously) if he really thought Bullet would still be here by the next snowfall. He was still here, not only for the entire next winter, but for the next four winters!

BE STRONG!

You'll need to be strong—for your dog's benefit and your own. We each have a different method of fortifying ourselves emotionally. When you're feeling overwhelmed or emotionally exhausted, gather strength from talking to family and friends about your journey. Make use of your support system. Take a break from researching. Sit by your dog and do nothing but stroke him for a while. If you're a "Type-A" personality, you might prefer to do more research to further verify that the home-care methods you choose have been successful with other dogs.

When it comes to death and dying, dogs are blessed with ignorance. They don't know that they may die soon or that they have a disease called cancer. Dogs don't regret or complain about what happened yesterday, nor do they anticipate or fear what might occur tomorrow.

Humans are not so lucky. We know, we fear, we anticipate and we project. While caring for your cancer-dog, shed your natural human inclination to dwell on these emotions, to fret over yesterday's decisions or worry about what tomorrow will bring. Be in the moment...Emulate your dog!

Maintaining this attitude adjustment may be an ongoing process. Every time Bullet went through a bad spell—and there were many—I wondered if and hoped that he was going to be able to recover "this time." I kept reminding myself, over and over, to remain calm, treat the symptoms and hope for the best.

KEEP A LOG

If you're a journal writer, sharpen your pencil! If not, do your best to at least keep a simple list of notable events. The information in your log may very well save your dog from having to endure side effects unnecessarily. A few months into treatment, you may find yourself trying to remember, *"Which agent was it that prompted that terrible reaction?"* or, *"How long was it before my dog was feeling better the last time he had this reaction?"* or, *"What were his symptoms and which remedy was it that finally alleviated those symptoms?"*

Veterinarians that you consult during the course of your dog's treatment may ask you for information such as when you started giving your dog a particular medication or supplement, at what dose and how he responded to it. Your logbook will contain the answers and will help you to help the doctor make effective, fully informed recommendations.

Keep track of events during the course of treatment—simple notations made in a notebook could help you get a repeat episode under control quickly.

ITEMS TO INCLUDE IN YOUR LOG
- Medications and supplements given
- Any change in diet
- Any change in eating, urination and defecation habits
- Names and dates of treatments
- Side effects and reactions
- What attempts were made to counteract side effects
- What worked and what didn't
- How long it took for the remedy to resolve the problem
- Which team member (or other source) suggested the remedy
- Secondary illnesses

Ask your veterinarians for copies of blood test results, laboratory reports and surgery reports. Keep these in a file for easy reference.

DON'T BE AFRAID TO ASK

How much medical information do you want to hear? Some people find it all too complicated to understand, others would rather put the problem in the doctors' hands and leave it at that. As a result, many medical doctors and veterinarians comply. They tend not to volunteer extensive medical information and they don't expect their patients/clients to be interested or to participate in the decision-making process.

If "medicalese" is Greek to you and you want to keep it that way, you can ask your veterinarian to consult with a specialist—a board certified veterinary oncologist. Members of this small and elite group of highly trained experts are aware of the most up to date data about canine cancer care. With the assistance of your veterinarian and a well-placed specialist, you will design a solid treatment plan for your dog.

If you *do* want to know and you want to play a role in deciding on a treatment plan, make very sure that your veterinarian is aware of this. Don't passively nod "okay" when your veterinarian outlines a plan. Rather, ask him to outline all of the options and to explain why he chose the treatment plan that he did. Let your veterinarian know that, with his guidance, you will make all of the final decisions about your dog's care. Talk to other veterinarians, consult specialists and anyone you can think of who might be able to contribute to your knowledge bank about canine cancer. As your dog's first advocate, make the best decision you can and don't look back.

I was dreading the day Bullet would come out of remission. *How will I know? When might it be? What will happen next?* That feeling of being unprepared, of not knowing what to expect, was creating anxiety. The solution was to gather some information, a few statistics and some hard cold facts. So, I asked.

Dr. Porzio explained that Bullet's lymph nodes would quite suddenly become enlarged. *Might I miss it?* "Like golf balls," he said. He showed me exactly where these golf balls would appear and I started to check for lymph-node enlargement every day. I simply incorporated the check into my petting motion. Scratch the top of the head, tweak the ears, run my fingers down his back along the spine...And then add a quick but firm sweep of the hand over the locations where the nodes reside. I stopped the daily checks perhaps a year after the chemotherapy treatment plan was completed, but I still to this day do a check about once a week.

Dr. Porzio and I discussed various rescue therapies in current use for dogs relapsing after a remission. We agreed that if or when Bullet came out of remission, we would call on Dr. Ruslander, our board certified veterinary oncologist consultant, for guidance. We also discussed what would happen "at the end" and agreed on a course of action. Although morbid, the conversation gave me a comforting sense of preparedness.

Be very clear about what the signs will be if and when your dog comes out of remission. Ask your oncologist to show you exactly where you will see or feel a change and what it will look like. The first sign of a failed remission is often enlarged lymph nodes (see "Lymph Node Locator). Feel the nodes regularly and make a note of their sizes. Inform your doctor immediately if the nodes suddenly feel larger.

Apart from enlarged lymph nodes, Bullet was asymptomatic at the time of his diagnosis. During the year and a half that followed, I watched him become terribly ill many times. Each time, I found myself thinking, "Maybe there was a misdiagnosis and I'm putting Bullet through the agony of cancer treatment—perhaps killing him with it—

when he doesn't even have cancer!" The thought haunted me and I became more and more certain that Bullet actually didn't have cancer at all.

I asked Dr. Porzio and Dr. Hoskins, separately, about the possibility of a misdiagnosis. They each assured me that there was absolutely no chance of this and reminded me that the biopsy had been evaluated by two different diagnosticians. Their certainty saddened me as it pulled me out of my momentary (and hopeful) denial and forced me to face again that Bullet really did have cancer. At the

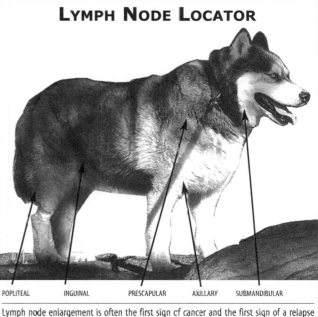

LYMPH NODE LOCATOR

POPLITEAL   INGUINAL   PRESCAPULAR   AXILLARY   SUBMANDIBULAR

Lymph node enlargement is often the first sign of cancer and the first sign of a relapse from a remission. Check your dog's lymph nodes regularly. (Of course, there's a matching set on left side of the dog.)

same time, it steeled me and reinforced my resolve to keep fighting without wondering if Bullet was suffering for no good reason.

READ, READ, READ

At this time, there are only a few books about canine cancer that are written for the layperson. If you're "online," you'll find that there's a wealth of information on the Internet. There, you can access a great deal of information quickly, including coverage of the most current theories about canine cancer treatment and about newly discovered cancer-fighting supplements. Always double-check the accuracy of information you garner from the Internet with your veterinarian (see "Resources on the Net," page 15).

Don't forget to listen to your dog! If you watch and listen closely, you may learn something about what he wants and what he needs. You may think he's capable of communicating only that he wants to eat or has to pee...but don't discount the possibility that he can say much more than that. Watch his facial expressions and his body language as well. For help understanding your dog's language, read *Dog Language: An Encyclopedia of Canine Behavior,* by Roger Abrantes.

"IT'S JUST A DOG!"

What *is* a dog's life worth? The typical family pet will not grow up, develop a career and contribute to society. He won't support you in your senior years or take care of you when you become feeble. He won't even bring you a cup of tea when you've got the flu. (My apologies to all search and rescue, seeing eye, seizure alert and other working dogs for this generalization.)

The typical pet dog *will* give unconditional love, loyalty and companionship. Indeed, he will devote his entire existence to the solitary purpose of pleasing the special person or persons in his life. In return, we give our dogs love, excellent care and respect.

With love, care and respect, we cancer-dog caretakers are forced to make some very difficult decisions about things like surgery, radiation therapy, chemotherapy, palliative care and euthanasia. None of these options are attractive. Each of the various responses is valid, so long as it comes from the heart and includes respect.

Are you committed to taking the journey through cancer treatment with your dog? If so, many will understand your decision. There are many people who will go to great lengths to care

RESOURCES ON THE NET

There's a wealth of information at your fingertips if you know how to find it. You might start by exploring the Web sites managed by veterinary schools. There you'll find information about research, treatment and clinical trials (see page 22).

There are many reliable resources on the net. A few are listed below.

GENERAL INFO WEB SITES

www.vetcancersociety.org
www.cancer.gov
www.morrisanimalfoundation.org
http://perseusfoundation.org/
www.avma.org
www.caninecancerawareness.com
www.gcvs.com/oncology
www.thensome.com
www.petcancer.htm
www.haileybell.homestead.com/

To search further, start with a search engine. My favorite is Copernic (www.Copernic.com). Whichever engine you choose, just rev it up and start to plug in words. It might take you a while and several combinations of words before you find what you're looking for—be patient. Use combinations of words that describe the thing about which you want information. Try "canine +cancer," "chemotherapy+dogs," or "veterinary +oncology." From the Web sites listed in the search results, explore any that look as though they might be helpful. If one's not helpful, close it and go on to the next Web site in the list.

At each Web site, you'll find "links." Links are usually blue and underlined. Click on any links that look promising or pique your interest. Save good Web sites as "bookmarks" or "favorites," or print out important pages during your search. As you branch off from Web site to Web site and click from link to link, you will eventually and inevitably forget where you started.

You can also use a search engine to research medications and treatments, supplements, clinical trials and diets for canine cancer or for a particular type of canine cancer. If you hear of a supplement that might help your dog, open your search engine and type in its name to search for information about it.

The Internet can be a wonderful resource, but be forewarned: Some of the information you come across may not be accurate. Always check the source and validity of information that you find on the net before adding it to your treatment plan.

E-GROUPS

Online support groups for people with cancer-dogs are very effective. There's a circular dynamic apparent within these groups: A distraught newcomer posts an urgent plea for help and receives mountains of information and loving support. Before long, the new member has the knowledge and experience needed to become a teacher and supporter of the next rash of new members who are posting urgent pleas for help.

E-groups devoted to pet cancer are listed below. You can participate or just read the questions, answers and advice posted by others.

http://forums.delphiforums.com/ petcancer
http://groups.yahoo.com/group/ caninecancercomfort
http://groups.yahoo.com/group/ CanineCancerAwareness
http://groups.yahoo.com/group/ endlesslove

for and provide medical treatment for a beloved dog. It's not unheard of for a caretaker to refinance a home in order to be able to pay for canine cancer treatment. I've also spoken to caretakers who were able to take a leave of absence from work in order to care for their cancer-dogs.

And then there are those others, who will not be able to understand. Prepare yourself to hear from those around you who are not devout dog lovers, "But it's just a dog!" Don't allow the naysayers to sway you, but don't think for a moment that you will sway them. At best, you'll convince them that you're entitled to your (nutty) beliefs about the value of a dog's life.

Whether you decide to shore up your resources and marshal your forces for the long haul or to release your pet through euthanasia in order to save him from suffering, make peace with your decision and enact it with love and with great respect for your dog.

NINE STEPS

Barbara Brandon, author of *Survive Your Cancer: The Essential Who, What, Where, When & How Guide for Cancer Patients & Their Families*, provides a list of actions for cancer patients to take. These actions are parallel to those that you, as your dog's advocate, will take on his behalf.

1. Talk about your cancer
2. Get on the internet or get to a library
3. Find the top treatment facilities
4. Change your fears into questions
5. Use the proper medical terminology
6. Obtain your medical records
7. Write your own medical history
8. Be direct and persistent
9. Trust your instincts

Reprinted by permission of Barbara Brandon

EARLY DECISIONS

When cancer is suspected, the first task is to establish a diagnosis. A veterinarian may be able to establish a preliminary diagnosis of a mass or tumor with some degree of certainty based only on observation and a hands-on examination. A definitive diagnosis, however, is necessary in order for the doctor to formulate a prognosis and determine what type of treatment is appropriate. Dr. Ruslander points out that it's a good idea to seek out a second opinion and an alternate interpretation of test results when there's any possibility of a misdiagnosis.

A diagnosis can be ascertained in several ways. Often, a diagnosis is based on the results of a fine-needle aspirate biopsy. If you can feel the mass with your fingers, a needle biopsy will probably be attempted. This is because a needle biopsy is less invasive, less traumatic and less expensive than a surgical biopsy. It's is a simple procedure, generally done without any need for anesthesia. Fluid or tissue cells extracted from the mass through a needle are studied under a microscope to determine if cancer is present. The procedure is unsuccessful if lymph fluid is not extracted.

When a needle biopsy fails to render a diagnosis, a surgical biopsy is performed and the type of cancer and stage are reported. If a surgical biopsy is required, consider having an oncologist confer with your veterinarian beforehand. In some cases, the tumor can be removed during a biopsy procedure without the need for a second operation—but only if all cancer cells in the proximity of the tumor are removed, achieving "clean margins." This requires tissue testing during the procedure and the specialized equipment needed is generally found only in the clinic of a veterinary oncologist.

In some cases, a diagnosis is made via imaging technology such as ultrasound, radiography (x-ray) or nuclear scintigraphy (bone scan). Tumors in the brain or spinal cord, for example, are often diagnosed via magnetic resonance imaging (MRI) because they are difficult to access by any other method and surgery in these areas is too radical a procedure to obtain a preliminary diagnosis.

TREATMENT DECISIONS

If your veterinarian concludes that your dog has cancer, he may then refer you to a specialist in veterinary cancer—a veterinary oncologist. The specialist will examine your dog, review his medical history and recommend a treatment plan. If there's no reasonable hope of treatment success, the veterinarian may recommend palliative care. This type of treatment does not aim to cure or

NO CONTRACT

A decision to begin cancer treatment for your dog does not in any way obligate you to continue treatment ad infinitum. When making this decision, keep in mind that there is no contract—you can stop treatment at any time.

It's always difficult to call it quits, but it's even more difficult to keep an unhappy animal alive when there's no real hope for a turnaround. A decline in the dog's quality of life is always a good and compelling reason to stop treatment.

People often discontinue cancer treatment because their dog isn't responding to treatment or becomes dangerously ill from it. Others stop due to financial constraints.

There's nothing wrong with giving your dog an extra 3, 5 or 7 months of life (and also giving yourself those additional months to spend with him) and then choosing a stopping point when the financial outlay has reached a certain limit.

Take the pressure off! If you're unable to make a long-term decision, keep your options open by providing treatment until you're able to decide. If you withhold treatment and later decide to treat, the time lost may diminish the chances of success.

fight the cancer. It aims to maximize your pet's comfort level and quality of life in his time remaining and perhaps, with luck, to prolong that period of time.

Your first decision is whether or not to go ahead with treatment. Declining treatment, you can simply enjoy the time you have left with your dog and let nature take its course. A decision to decline medical treatment doesn't mean that there's nothing you can do. You can help your dog fight cancer and perhaps survive longer.

You may be able to buy some time, slow down the disease process and postpone the decline. Take the same dietary and supplemental measures employed by those who do opt for medical treatment. If you have decided to forgo traditional treatment but want to learn about dietary measures that are known to benefit cancer patients, see Chapter 7. For information about supplements that may improve your dog's quality of life and perhaps prolong his life, skip to Chapter 8.

If you decide to treat the cancer aggressively, the course of action may be clear. There may be only one type of treatment that's effective for the type of cancer that your dog has. Often, there is no clear treatment of choice; no definitive results from experiments showing that one particular course of action has the best chance of success.

If you don't have time or if you have a limited understanding of medicine but want the best chance of treatment success, consult several experts in canine cancer and then make an informed decision based on their cumulative recommendations. You can be an active participant in the decision-making process for your dog's treatment without having a degree in veterinary medicine.

When a treatment is recommended, seek out a second opinion. You might want to seek out a third if the first two conflict. Very often, a doctor will recommend the treatment with which he is most familiar. It may or may not be the treatment that will be most effective for your dog. Make use of the consultation services that are offered by many veterinary oncologists in private practice and at the schools of veterinary medicine.

Your veterinarian and any consultants that you enlist will help you to determine what your options are, depending on the type of cancer, its stage and grade and the overall health of your dog. You have now taken the first step toward assembling your team. *"What team,"* you ask? You're going to launch an offensive against your dog's cancer and it will involve a larger cast than just you, your dog and a veterinarian (see "Assemble Your Team," page 20).

ASSEMBLE YOUR TEAM

The size and scope of your team is entirely up to you—you are the captain of the team. Don't be afraid to add to and redefine your team roster. You should have complete and implicit confidence in each of your practitioners and consultants. Each of your team members must have expert knowledge in the facet of cancer treatment to which they are going to contribute to your dog's treatment or care, and they should be invested in seeing your dog survive with a good quality of life.

▶ **Your veterinarian,** who knows your dog's personality and medical history better than any other member of your team. Some general practice veterinarians provide cancer treatment in addition to running a general practice. Keep in mind that these doctors devote a fraction of their time to cancer treatment, whereas a specialist has a great deal more experience in treating canine cancer.

▶ **A board certified veterinary oncologist** at a veterinary school or major veterinary hospital is an essential member of the team. This specialist has access to cutting edge information and news of experimental treatments not yet in general use. He may provide your dog's treatment or act as a consultant to the veterinarian providing treatment. As a consultant, he'll be available for consultation when necessary throughout the course of treatment.

The doctor providing cancer treatment, whether a general practice veterinarian or a veterinary oncologist, will be a central clearinghouse for information. He'll provide test results and progress reports to you and to other members of your team when appropriate.

▶ **A holistic veterinarian.** Holistic veterinary medicine can enhance and supplement traditional treatments. If you forgo traditional treatment entirely, a holistic veterinarian can serve as your dog's primary doctor.

If your general practice veterinarian is holistic, find an allopathic (traditional) team member so that you'll be able to receive input from both camps.

Some holistic veterinarians are "purists" and will refuse to treat your dog if he is undergoing traditional treatment. Likewise, some traditional veterinarians will refuse to treat your dog if you employ certain holistic methods. If you wish to use a combination of holistic and traditional therapies as I have, you'll need to find open-minded team members.

▶ **Specialists,** as needed, to treat secondary or unrelated health problems that arise. Any team member can refer you to appropriate specialists. All specialists must be informed of your dog's cancer status and treatment.

▶ **Other caretakers of dogs with cancer:** Your veterinarian may put you in touch with one of his other clients or you may already know someone fitting this description. A great deal of information-sharing between caretakers of dogs with cancer takes place on the Internet (see "Resources on the Net," page 15).

▶ For dogs with cancer requiring radiation therapy and/or surgery, Dr. Ruslander recommends that the caretaker add to this team roster a board certified radiation oncologist and/or a board certified surgeon, accordingly.

CHOOSING A DOCTOR

Currently, there are about 150 board certified veterinary oncologists in the U.S. To earn this title, veterinarians complete a minimum of two to three years of rigorous clinical experience and training in veterinary oncology and must pass a two-day theoretical and practical examination.

A board certified veterinary oncologist should be included as a member of your team. Because there are (in the U.S.) hundreds of thousands of dogs with various cancers at any given time and only 150 oncologists, it's not possible for every cancer-dog to be treated by an oncologist. According to Dr. Hoskins,

> More and more general practice veterinarians are acquiring telemedicine equipment. Using this equipment, digital X-ray and ultrasound images are generated on-site and sent via cable modem to a specialist anywhere in the world for interpretation and consultation.

In November 2002, Bullet developed a heart condition and we took advantage of telemedicine capabilities. Electrocardiograms (EKGs) were performed on Bullet in Dr. Hoskin's general practice clinic, with no cardiologist on staff. Bullet's EKG signals are transmitted by telephone directly to Cardiopet. Veterinary cardiologists interpret the results and a report is faxed to the clinic within 24 hours (or sooner, for an additional fee), along with a prognosis and treatment recommendations.

Oncura Partners™ is the oncological equivalent of Cardiopet, providing expert consultation and guidance to general practice veterinarians who treat cancer in dogs, cats and other animals. Most "GP" veterinarians who treat cancer do so in addition to annual check-ups, emergency procedures, spays and neuters. It's important to include in your team a specialist in veterinary oncology, who devotes his full attention to cancer treatment.

A veterinary oncologist could be your dog's primary cancer treatment provider, or may serve as a consultant. Three factors will decide which of these roles a board certified veterinary oncologist plays on your team. Proximity (there may not be a veterinary oncologist near you); cost (a board certified oncologist's fees will be higher than your veterinarian's) and familiarity (important if your dog is fearful of new people). If necessary, you can find a general practice veterinarian or one who's board certified in internal medicine to provide cancer treatment and also enlist a board certified veterinary oncologist to consult and make treatment recommendations.

SCHOOLS OF VETERINARY MEDICINE

SCHOOL	PHONE	WEBSITE
Auburn University	(334) 844-2685	www.vetmed.auburn.edu
University of California-Davis	(530) 752-1360	www.vetmed.ucdavis.edu
Colorado State University	(303) 491-7051	www.cvmbs.colostate.edu
Cornell University	(607) 253-3060	www.vet.cornell.edu
University of Florida	(904) 392-4700	www.vetmed.ufl.edu
University of Georgia	(706) 542-3461	www.vet.uga.edu
University of Illinois-Urbana	(217) 333-2760	www.cvm.uiuc.edu
Iowa State University	(515) 294-1242	www.vetmed.iastate.edu
Kansas State University	(785) 532-6011	www.vet.ksu.edu
Louisiana State University	(225) 346-3100	www.vetmed.lsu.edu
Michigan State University	(517) 355-6509	http://cvm.vsu.edu
University of Minnesota	(612) 624-9227	www.cvm.umn.edu
Mississippi State University	(662) 325-3432	www.cvm.msstate.edu
University of Missouri	(573) 882-3877	www.cvm.missouri.edu
North Carolina State University	(919) 513-6200	www.cvm.ncsu.edu
Ohio State University	(614) 292-1171	www.vet.ohio-state.edu
Oklahoma State University	(405) 744-6648	www.cvm.okstate.edu
Oregon State University	(541) 737-2141	www.vet.orst.edu
University of Pennsylvania	(215) 898-5434	www.vet.upenn.edu
Purdue University	(765) 494-7607	www.vet.purdue.edu
University of Tennessee	(865) 974-7262	www.vet.utk.edu
Texas A&M University	(409) 845-5051	www.cvm.tamu.edu
Tufts University	(508) 839-5302	www.tufts.edu/vet
Tuskegee University	(334) 727-8173	http://svmc107.tusk.edu
Virginia-Maryland Regional College of Veterinary Medicine	(540) 231-4621	www.vetmed.vt.edu
Washington State University	(509) 335-9515	www.vetmed.wsu.edu
Western University	(909) 469-5628	www.westernu.edu/cym.html
University of Wisconsin-Madison	(608) 263-6716	www.vetmed.wisc.edu

Many oncologists at Veterinary Schools or in private practice assist veterinarians treating cancer dogs. Your veterinarian can arrange for a phone consultation. The specialist will review your dog's laboratory reports and diagnostic tests before the consultation. Most consultants prefer to speak directly with the veterinarian rather than to the caretaker.

To find a board certified veterinary oncologist, contact the veterinary school nearest to you (see page 22) or the American College of Veterinary Internal Medicine (ACVIM). At [www.acvim.org], click "Diplomates" and "Oncology." Select the geographic listing.

If you choose an oncology consultant whose office is nearby, make an appointment at some point during the course of treatment so that he can meet your dog in the flesh (or "in the fur"). If the consultant you choose is not nearby, however, don't fret. A face-to-face meeting is preferable but is not necessary. Once the treatment plan is in place, your doctor will send copies of pertinent reports, tests and findings to the consultant and contact him whenever a decision needs to be made. You may at any time ask your doctor to consult a specialist.

To find a holistic veterinarian in your area, see Web site: [http://ahvma.org/referral/index.html]

or call (410) 569-0795. If you need help finding an oncology radiologist, you'll find help at Web site: [www.vetcancersociety.org/pdf/radiation.pdf].

To Test or not To Test

During the diagnosis stage, your veterinarian most likely did some bloodwork and either a fine-needle aspirate biopsy or a surgical biopsy. There's no getting around the fact that initial diagnostics are necessary. From this point on, however, you will probably want to discuss the expected results and potential benefits of any recommended test. Discuss the typical discomfort, pain level or trauma and costs as well. If, in your mind, the potential benefits do not outweigh the potential distress or pain, "Just say no."

Anesthetics are poisons. Any test that requires anesthesia should be declined unless the results might contribute significant information about your dog's status that will determine what treatment or medication will be most effective.

At the time of Bullet's first chemotherapy treatment, two tests were suggested. The first was a bone marrow test. When I asked what purpose it would serve, Dr. Porzio explained that it would give us an idea of how advanced the cancer was.

Might the results alter Bullet's treatment? *"Not at all."* In other words, the result of this test would only allow the doctor to fine-tune the prognosis so that I would be able to make a note in my date book on the day that Bullet was expected to come out of remission. Because this procedure could be painful for the patient and not at all beneficial to him, I declined to have this test done.

CONSIDERATIONS FOR TREATMENT

▸ **The Age and Health of Your Dog.** In a geriatric dog, we must ask if the treatment is painful or traumatic for the dog. If so, how likely is it that after enduring the treatment, the dog's life will be extended appreciably? A dog of any age with preexisting medical issues may not tolerate treatment well and a preexisting condition may decrease the probability of success. Consider a treatment option that is less traumatic for the dog, even if it has a somewhat lower success rate.

▸ **Quality of Life.** How will treatment affect your dog's quality of life? The chances for treatment success must be weighed against the possibility and degree of trauma that your dog may endure from the treatment itself. There are many factors to weight and there is no right answer here, except the one that comes from your heart.

▸ **Input from Friends and Family.** Seek advice from people who value the life of a dog as highly as you do; people who will help you make a decision that's comfortable for you and right for your dog.

▸ **Gut Instincts.** Evaluate your dog's stamina and ability to endure medical interventions. Think about your own as well. If you have a strong suspicion that medical intervention will not be successful, you may choose to forgo treatment. Take your own psychological makeup into account as well. Are you prepared to roll up your sleeves, clean up vomit and diarrhea and possibly watch your dog endure periods of illness during treatment?

▸ **Financial Considerations.** Thinking of finances when making this decision is difficult emotionally. Are you putting a price on your dog's life? How much time will $1,000 buy him? How much money is it worth to keep him alive three more months? Two years? If you don't spend the money to keep him alive, will you regret it? If you do and the treatment isn't successful, will you regret having spent the money?

▸ **Be Decisive.** Make a decision that will not result in the birth of a haunting voice saying "I should have," or "I shouldn't have." Make the best decision that you can and then decide to accept, regardless of the outcome, that it was the best decision. If you have health insurance for your dog, great! Calculate the extent and scope of coverage so that there won't be any surprises later. If not, you may want to look into policies for your other pets, remembering that 50 percent of our cats and dog will have cancer in their lifetimes.

The second test that was suggested was an ultrasound on Bullet's heart. The chemotherapy agent that was going to be used was doxorubicin, which is highly cardiotoxic and should not be given if the animal's heart function is not strong enough to tolerate it. I gave this test a go-ahead.

Don't passively agree to all tests, but don't summarily reject all tests. Gather information and weed out all tests that are not going to benefit your dog. Of the tests that might benefit him, you will take on the difficult task of weighing trauma and expense against benefit. Will the test be traumatic for your dog? What are the chances that it will provide information that will benefit your dog by altering or fine-tuning his treatment plan and to what degree might it benefit him? It's not an easy task, but think it through, seek out the advice of your expert team members and make the best decision you can.

To Treat or Not to Treat

Deciding whether or not to treat a dog with cancer can be very difficult. If you're unable to make the decision right away, give some thought to the factors discussed in "Considerations for Treatment," page 24.

Think through all of the options. Clarify your feelings and thoughts about each and the reasons you might have for choosing or not choosing each option. Once you've made a decision, try not to second-guess yourself. Remember that there's no way of knowing what the outcome would have been had you chosen differently. Believe that the decision you made was for the best.

If you decide to treat your dog's cancer but the treatment isn't successful, will you have made the wrong choice? Of course not. If you don't treat or if you stop treatment and your dog perishes, don't torture yourself wondering whether or not your dog might have rebounded had you continued.

Some of the most difficult decisions that you'll have to make are whether or not to treat at all, which treatment to employ and when (if ever) to stop treatment. Here are some pointed questions that you can ask any member or all members of your team. Learning the answers may enable you to make these decisions with confidence.

QUESTIONS TO ASK YOUR VETERINARIAN

‣ What's the best possible outcome (i.e., cure; remission) of this treatment? How often is the "best possible outcome" achieved in dogs and in a dog the age and breed of my dog? What studies or tests were done to find this statistic?

- How invasive/traumatic would the treatment be for my dog?
- What's the worst possible outcome? Is it that the treatment simply fails to work or might my dog have adverse reactions? If so, what are the most common adverse reactions?
- If the treatment isn't successful, what is Plan B? (You'll ask these same questions about Plan B.)
- What costs are involved (long term) if Plan A works? If it doesn't work? Ask the same questions about Plan B, etc.
- What would you do if this were your dog?

Since you are your dog's first advocate and you are deciding on his behalf, imagine what you would choose if you were in his place. If you were diagnosed with cancer and were given the options that the veterinarians have outlined for your dog, what would you choose? Would you undergo any and all treatments that might grant you another month? Another year? If the treatment were painful, would that alter your decision?

Financial considerations are often the deciding factor in choosing treatment options for dogs with cancer. In light of the high incidence of canine cancer and the many other illnesses a dog can suffer, I encourage pet caretakers to purchase a medical insurance or discount program for their pets when they are young and healthy.

Bullet's insurance policy carrier, Veterinary Pet Insurance Co. (VPI), covered a great deal of the expense involved in Bullet's treatment. VPI has been thorough and fair in assessing claims and has always paid promptly. There are a number of companies that offer either medical insurance or discount programs for veterinary care. Research online or at the library to discover which policy will work best for your particular circumstances.

The Magic Bullet Fund, operating under the Perseus Foundation, is being created to provide assistance to caretakers who cannot afford to pay for treatment for their dogs. See page 109 for more information if you need assistance of if you are able to make a donation.

ABOUT CANINE CANCER

A 1999 survey conducted by American Pet Association Polls revealed that at that time there were more than 61 million pet dogs in the United States.[1] Fifty percent of our dogs will have some type of cancer in their lifetimes. This is a widely accepted estimate in veterinary oncology. If accurate, this means that 30 million of the dogs that are now in our homes and our hearts are destined to be diagnosed with cancer.

The Animal Cancer Institute provides a different statistic. It estimates the number of canine cancer cases diagnosed each year as follows: "Using crude estimates of cancer incidence, there are roughly 4 million new cancer diagnoses in dogs...made each year."[2]

Interestingly, the American Cancer Society states in a report called "Cancer Statistics 2003" that the risk of an American man developing cancer over his lifetime is one in two and that approximately one in three women in the United States will develop cancer over her lifetime.[3]

The most prevalent canine cancers are the various types of skin cancer (lumps and bumps in or under the skin), occurring at a rate of 450 per 100,000 dogs per year.[4] This means that approximately 274,000 dogs are diagnosed with skin cancer each year. These tumors are often benign (e.g., lipomas) but can be malignant (e.g., mast cell tumors), so a specific diagnosis is always necessary to determine the best treatment plan.

A veterinarian or veterinary oncologist may make a preliminary diagnosis by visual examination or palpation. A fine-needle aspirate or surgical biopsy will yield a definitive diagnosis and thus enable your veterinarian to recommend the best treatment plan.

The second most common canine cancer is mammary cancer. Mammary cancer is the most common malignant tumor in dogs. Mammary tumors occur at a rate of approximately 160 per 100,000 dogs in the population. This means that each year about 97,000 dogs are diagnosed with mammary cancer in the United States.

Of all canine mammary cancer cases, ninety-nine percent are females. The risk for intact females is 26 percent; for those spayed after the first heat cycle, 8 percent and those spayed before the first heat 0.05 percent.[5] In light of these statistics, it very difficult to justify *not* spaying a dog.

Third in line is lymphosarcoma (lymphoma). Philip Bergman, DVM, MS, PhD, ACVIM at the Bobst Animal Medical Center in New York, NY says, "Lymphoma is the third most common cancer found in dogs, with an incidence of 24 cases per 100,000 dogs per year."[6] Using the American Pet Association's 1999 estimate of 61 million dogs in the States, we find that more than 14,600 dogs in the U.S. alone are diagnosed with lymphoma each year. Another recent estimate is even more dismal: "A more recent report suggests an overall annual incidence [of canine lymphoma] approaching 110 cases per 100,000 [dogs].[7]

Although lymphoma in humans may be Hodgkin's or Non-Hodgkin's Lymphoma (NHL), canine lymphoma is always the malignant Non-Hodgkin's type. Non-Hodgkin's lympoma is sometimes abbreviated by veterinarians as LSA (lymphosarcoma).

A statistic from the *Veterinary Medical Data Base Program* (VMDP) at Purdue University reflects a gradual and consistent increase in the incidence of lymphoma between 1987 and 1997. At the starting point of this study, 0.75 percent of the dogs seen at 20 veterinary institutions had lymphoma. Ten years later, when the study was repeated, 2.0 percent had lymphoma.[8]

WHY DOGS GET CANCER

Why has there been such a sharp increase in the incidence of canine cancer? There are the obvious answers: Today's average caretaker is more knowledgeable and diligent about responsible pet care than ever before. It follows that our dogs are living longer, thus giving cancer a larger window

THE MOST COMMON CANINE CANCERS

Cutaneous Cancers
(Skin cancer; "lumps and bumps")

Adenocarcinoma
(Mammary Cancer)

Lymphosarcoma
(Lymphoma)

Cutaneous Cancers

- About 30 percent of all tumors in dogs are tumors of the skin or subcutaneous tumors.
- Of these, 70-80 percent are benign; the rest are malignant. About 20 percent of these are Mast Cell Tumors (MCTs).
- When possible, MCTs are surgically removed. If cancer cells remain, a second excision or radiation therapy is provided.
- If excision isn't possible, radiation therapy is used. About 60 percent of grade I and II MCTs are cured with radiation therapy alone.
- Surgery followed by multi-agent chemotherapy increases treatment success significantly. Single-agent chemotherapy with prednisone does not.
- In metastatic MCT's (Systemic Mast Cell Disease, SMCD), cure is rare. Chemotherapy (usually in the form of prednisone) is commonly used for palliative care.
- Breeds Predisposed for Mast Cell Tumors: Mixed breed dogs, Boxers, Boston Terriers, Labrador Retrievers, Beagles, Schnauzers.

Adenocarcinoma

- Mammary cancer is rare in male dogs. Of all cancerous tumors in females, 50 percent are mammary tumors.
- Half of all mammary tumors in female dogs are benign. These may become malignant if not removed.
- Of malignant mammary tumors, most are adenocarcinomas. The rest are inflammatory carcinomas, sarcomas and carcinosarcomas.
- Spaying female dogs before $1\frac{1}{2}$ years of age is protective against this cancer.
- Adenocarcinomas are removed with abnormal lymph nodes in the area.
- A mastectomy is performed if the tissue outside of the nodule is found to contain cancerous cells.
- The prognosis is good if the tumor is self-contained and excised. Prognosis worsens according to the extent that cancer cells have metastasized (spread) or invaded blood or lymphatic vessels.
- Breeds Predisposed: Several spaniel breeds, possibly the Poodle and the Dachshund.

Lymphosarcoma

- Of all lymphomas in dogs, 80 percent are multicentric. Average survival: 4 to 6 weeks without chemotherapy and 6 to 11 months with chemotherapy.
- With chemotherapy, 80 percent achieve remission quickly.
- Relapses are treated with reinduction or second-line chemotherapy. Each subsequent remission tends to be shorter in duration.
- Other common lymphomas: Mediastinal (the chest cavity—causes coughing, eventually inhibits the dog's ability to breathe); alimentary (gastrointestinal—causes vomiting, diarrhea, weight loss); cutaneous and ocular, lymphomas of central nervous system, kidney and bone.
- Solitary cutaneous lymphoma tumors may be treated surgically or with radiation therapy followed by chemotherapy. Diffuse tumors are treated with chemotherapy.
- Breeds Predisposed: Golden Retrievers, Cocker Spaniels, Rottweilers, Boxers, Basset Hounds, St. Bernards, Scottish Terriers, Airedale Terriers, English Bulldogs.

*All statistics are approximate and refer to canine cancers.[9]

of opportunity in which to strike...Advances in diagnostic testing in the world of veterinary medicine have made it possible to diagnose canine cancer earlier and with more clarity...Veterinary cancer treatment is more accessible and more successful than ever before, giving caretakers good reason to pursue a definitive diagnosis.

These arguments may explain some increase in the number of canine cancer cases diagnosed, but there's more to it than this. In *Natural Health Bible for Dogs & Cats*, Shawn Messonnier, DVM, discusses the causes of canine cancer and points to toxins (e.g., chemicals and food additives), vaccinations, genetics and aging.[10] Two factors are generally accepted to be causative in canine cancer: 1) Exposure to lawn chemicals is the primary cause of lymphoma in dogs and 2) Obesity leads to canine bladder cancer. "Second-hand smoke" is suspected but to date has not been documented to be a cause of cancer in dogs.

LAWN-CARE PRODUCTS

Lawn-care products, including fertilizers, weed killers (herbicides) and pesticides are thought to be the number one causative factor of canine lymphoma. A 2003 study conducted at Purdue University School of Veterinary Medicine concluded the following:

"The risk of transitional cell carcinoma (TCC) was significantly increased among dogs exposed to lawns or gardens treated with both herbicides and insecticides or with herbicides alone. Dogs exposed to lawns or gardens treated with insecticides alone had a small, but not significantly, increased risk of TCC compared with dogs exposed to untreated lawns."[11]

Manufacturers of toxic lawn-care products generally recommend that pets be kept off of a newly treated lawn for 24 hours after application, but this may not be a strong enough warning. Chemicals picked up outdoors on the soles of our shoes or bare feet do not end up in our mouths—most of us don't lick the bottoms of our shoes or feet (at least I don't). But Bullet does and, most likely, your dog does too.

Even if you use organic, natural lawn-care products, the products a neighbor uses on his lawn can easily be blown onto your yard. In spite of all of your precautions, your dog still winds up licking those harmful chemicals off of his feet.

Pesticides that we spray on our bodies are generally labeled "not for internal use." Be aware that if you use bug spray on your arm and your dog licks it, he is in effect "using it internally." For alternative nontoxic lawn care ideas, see article

"Ten Simple Steps to Ecological Lawn Care."[12] Nontoxic lawn care products are offered by companies such as Home Harvest Garden Supply, Inc.,[13] Peaceful Valley Farm Supply[14] and others.

HOUSEHOLD CLEANING PRODUCTS

Floor-polishing, carpet-cleaning and oven-cleaning products often contain chemicals that cause cancer (carcinogens). We are a chemical-happy society but many chemicals that we use are entirely unnecessary. For example, cleaning the kitchen floor can be accomplished with squeaky-clean results using hot water mixed with a mild, natural soap. Any stubborn dirt that remains can be cleaned more aggressively with a stronger cleanser and then rinsed thoroughly.

For in-depth information about safe house-cleaning and gardening practices, visit the Web site of Ernestina Parziale, Certified Herbalist: [http://earthnotes.tripod.com/clnrecipes.htm].

FOOD

If chemicals in the environment cause cancer, what about pesticides that are used on fruits and vegetables? What about antibiotics and growth hormones that are injected into food animals and dyes used to make foods more appealing? Could genetically engineered food products also cause cancer? You've undoubtedly heard these questions raised about the food that you eat and they are equally relevant to the food that your dog eats.

Because diet plays a role in the fight against cancer, it follows that diet would also be capable of preventing or causing cancer. According to Ann N. Martin, author of *Food Pets Die For*, "Many of the grains used in commercial pet food contain levels of herbicides, pesticides, and fungicides that are cancer-causing agents."[15] The author explains that although these grains didn't pass inspection for use in human foods, they were deemed adequate for use in pet foods.

Dr. Messonnier says, "Various food additives have also demonstrated carcinogenic activity in laboratory animals, prompting many owners to prepare food at home or select diets that do not contain these synthetic additives and preservatives."[16]

For more information about the causes of cancer in companion animals, read *Why Is Cancer Killing Our Pets?* by Deborah Straw and for more information on toxins to dogs, contact the ASPCA's Animal Poison Control Center.

VACCINES

The administration of annual vaccinations to dogs has been suspected by some veterinarians to be a causative factor in the growing number of canine cancer diagnoses. In other words, vaccinations that are given to our dogs to protect them from a variety of ills may cause cancer. Cancer that develops due to vaccination is called Vaccinosis or Vaccine Associated Sarcoma and usually takes the form of a tumor at the vaccination site. Vaccinosis is more common in cats than in dogs.

Holistically-minded veterinary practitioners are generally against the general administration of annual vaccinations. Many question this practice based on the fact that vaccines given to people are generally effective for many years. They are not repeated annually.

In fact, in April of 2001, the Executive Board of the American Veterinary Medical Association (AVMA) issued the following statement:

> There is evidence that some vaccines provide immunity beyond one year. Revaccination of patients with sufficient immunity does not add measurably to their disease resistance, and may increase their risk of adverse post-vaccination events.[17]

Veterinarians subscribing to a more traditional school of thought remind us of epidemics that have been avoided or curtailed and about the thousands of canine lives that have been spared by the advent of the vaccine. They vaccinate their own pets. It doesn't make sense, they say, to risk losing a dog to a disease when there's a vaccine that can practically guarantee to safeguard him against it. This makes good sense if there is such a risk. Vaccinating a pet against a disease that is not a threat in the region where he lives, however, does not make good sense.

Whether or not to vaccinate a pet is up to the caretaker, with the exception of the rabies vaccine, which is required by law in some states. In order to decide which vaccines you want your healthy pet to have and which vaccines you want to decline, gather the following important pieces of information through research or simply by asking your veterinarian.

CONSIDERATIONS FOR VACCINATION

▸ What are the odds that your pet might contract the disease? What percent of pets in your region have it?
▸ What's the efficacy of the vaccine? In other words, to what degree is it successful in protecting pets from the disease?
▸ When a pet gets this disease, what is the treatment? Is it successful? Painful? Expensive?
▸ What's the overall prognosis for dogs who contract this disease?

If there's a low incidence of a particular disease in your region and the treatment for the disease is generally successful and not painful for your pet (or for you, monetarily), then the answer is not to vaccinate. At the other end of the spectrum, if there's a significant incidence of the disease in your region, it has dire medical consequences, there's no effective, safe and economically viable treatment, then the answer is to vaccinate.

In most cases, unfortunately, the answers are not this clear cut. There's no clear cut-off point at which the incidence is low enough and the treatment success rate's high enough to justify not taking preventive measures. The calculations become even fuzzier when we insert into the equation the question, "What negative effects might the preventive have on your dog?"

Weigh the risks of medicating against the risks of not medicating, research the incidence of the disease in your region and the efficacy of the preventive and then make your best decision. Many experts believe that an animal with cancer should not receive any vaccines at all. For information about vaccines and cancer, see pages 99 and 100.

CHEMICALS

The general proliferation of chemicals in the environment may be a causative factor in the increased incidence of canine cancer. Chemicals deemed safe for use by humans might harm, kill or cause cancer in a dog. Many products that we use regularly are carried to the ground by gravity after being used. These fumes and residues may not harm us, but we're not inhaling them in a highly concentrated form. A canine's nose and mouth are far closer to the ground than are ours, however, and he may inhale or ingest substances that don't harm us because they make contact with only the soles of our shoes.

Note that the word "nontoxic" on a product label generally means that the product is not harmful to the environment. It does not necessarily mean that it's safe for a dog to breathe, lick off the floor or lick off of his paws.

PREDISPOSITION BY BREED

Breed seems to be a factor in the incidence of canine cancer. Studies show that dogs of certain specific breeds are more likely to develop cancer than are others. Boxers and Golden Retrievers are at the top of this list. However, Dr. Ruslander points out, these statistics are not necessarily meaningful because many such studies are not well performed. "Since cancer is not a reportable disease," explains Dr. Ruslander, "we may be seeing a biased population." His meaning is that an unknown number of canine cancer cases are not diagnosed, and that if caretakers of certain breeds of dogs are more likely to pursue cancer diagnosis and treatment than caretakers of other breeds or of mixed-breed dogs, then the number of cases reported may not be a "meaningful" statistic.

References

1   The American Pet Association
    [www.apapets.com/petstats2.htm]

2   The Animal Cancer Institute
    [www.animalcancerinstitute.com/oncology.html]

3   "Cancer Statistics 2003 Script for Slide Presentation," The American Cancer Society. ACS Document Code #8641.03.

4   *Small Animal Clinical Oncology*, editors Stephen J. Withrow, DVM, diplomate ACVIM (oncology) and E. Gregory MacEwen, VMD, diplomate ACVIM (oncology and internal medicine). W.B. Saunders Company, 2001, p.233.

5   ibid, p.455.

6   *Animal News*, The Morris Animal Foundation. Volume III, 2001.

7   *Veterinary Oncology Secrets*, editor Robert C. Rosenthal, DVM, PhD. Hanley & Belfus, Inc, 2001, p.180.

8   *Small Animal Clinical Oncology*, p.558.

9   Data for this chart was collected from two sources: *Small Animal Clinical Oncology* and *Manual of Small Animal Internal Medicine*, by Richard W. Nelson, DVM and C. Guillermo Couto, DVM. Mosby, 1999.

10 *Natural Health Bible for Dogs & Cats,* by Shawn Messonnier, DVM. Prima Publishing, 2001, p.44.

11 *Journal of the American Veterinary Medical Association,* April 15, 2004.

12 "Ten Simple Steps to Ecological Lawn Care." *Natural Life Magazine,* May/June 1995, p.2.

13 Home Harvest Garden Supply, Inc.
    Phone: (800) 348-4769
    Website: [http://homeharvest.com]

14 Peaceful Valley Farm Supply
    Phone: (888) 784-1722
    Website: [www.groworganic.com]

15 *Food Pets Die For: Shocking Facts about Pet Food,* by Ann N. Martin. New Sage Press, 2003, p.9.

16 *Natural Health Bible for Dogs & Cats,* p.335.

17 A 2001 report by the American Veterinary Medical Association. Available online at:
    [www.avma.org/policies/vaccination.htm]

MEDICAL INTERVENTIONS

Before cancer treatment can begin, a definitive diagnosis is necessary. Different types of treatment are used for different types of cancer. The type, stage and grade of the cancer are all important factors and with this information, a veterinary oncologist determines which treatment plan will have the best chance of fighting that particular cancer.

Surgery, radiation therapy and chemotherapy are the medical interventions most commonly used to fight cancer in dogs (and people as well). Chemotherapy is effective in curing or managing certain types of canine cancer. Chemotherapy is the treatment of choice for canine multicentric lymphoma.

If chemotherapy is agreed upon, a protocol must be chosen (see "About Protocols," page 49). Statistics comparing the relative success rates of various protocols are readily available to veterinarians. They are updated periodically in order to keep the veterinary community apprised of new developments.

Chemotherapy is used to treat most types of canine cancer because, according to Dr. Porzio, "Many malignancies, including lymphoma, have already spread at the time of diagnosis. Hence the importance of chemotherapy with or without surgery." When a dog comes out of remission, "rescue" or "second line" or "reinduction" chemotherapy is attempted.

According to Dr. Ruslander, about 25 percent of dogs with multicentric lymphoma that are treated with chemotherapy survive for two years and approximately 5 to 10 percent achieve a "cure." When I asked what constitutes a "cure," Dr. Ruslander responded that there is a cure when the tumors do not return (enlarged lymph nodes are considered "tumors").

Kevin A. Hahn, DVM, PhD, diplomate ACVIM (Oncology) at Gulf Coast Veterinary Specialists in Houston, TX, says, "It's difficult to say that a dog with lymphoma is cured because you never stop looking for new tumors. But with ongoing treatment and observation, one-year and even two-year survivors are possible." See Chapter 5 for more information about chemotherapy.

DIAGNOSTICS

When a veterinarian suspects that a dog has cancer, he'll palpate the lump or enlarged lymph node and attempt a fine-needle aspirate biopsy. If a diagnosis can't be made using this method, a surgical biopsy or an ultrasound-guided biopsy is performed to definitively rule out or diagnose cancer. In this case, surgery serves a diagnostic purpose. During the surgical biopsy, a lump or tumor may be removed. If it's found to be cancerous, further treatment is almost always recommended. It's a good idea to consult with a veterinary oncologist before a surgical biopsy is performed because suspicion of certain types of cancer alters the surgical procedure.

SURGICAL INTERVENTIONS

After a diagnosis has been made, surgery may be recommended as part of the treatment plan. Surgery can serve a curative or a palliative role in cancer treatment. Curative surgery involves the removal of a tumor or a lymph node in an attempt to slow the spread of or entirely remove the cancer. Says Dr. Porzio, "Curative surgery involving the removal of a cancerous tumor is generally followed by chemotherapy in order to eradicate stray cancer cells that may remain."

Palliative measures are not intended to cure but rather to reduce a dog's pain and/or improve his mobility and quality of life while the cancer runs its course. Debulking (cytoreductive surgery) of a large tumor is often intended to make a dog more comfortable.

When cure is the goal, every effort is made to remove the entire tumor and surrounding tissue as well. The incomplete removal of a tumor is a common type of palliative surgery. The trauma of major surgery is avoided while improving quality of life and perhaps prolonging life.

RADIATION THERAPY

Radiation can be very effective in treating tumors. Periodically, for several weeks or more, the tumored part of the dog's body is exposed to carefully controlled doses of radiation. This is often used in conjunction with surgery or chemotherapy, depending on the type, stage and location of the tumor.

Radiation therapy is also considered a viable alternative to the amputation of a tumored limb. Amputation offers a higher certainty that the cancer has been eradicated, and most dogs adjust quite well after a single-limb amputation. However, some tumor types respond well to radiation therapy and some caretakers are reluctant to subject their dog to amputation surgery.

Half-body Irradiation (HBI) is a treatment in clinical trials for dogs with lymphoma. Dr. Ruslander reports that this is used at NCSU but adds that no final conclusion has been drawn on the success of this treatment modality. In Dr. Rus-

lander's words, "The jury's still out about HBI."

Radiation therapy is not without side effects. In the book, *Pets Living With Cancer*, author Robin Downing, DVM, discusses side effects common when radiation is applied to the head. These are faucitis mucositis (an inflammation of the tissue lining the mouth) and dry eye (irritation of tissue around the eyes with decreased tear production). Dr. Downing writes about desquamation of the skin around any radiated area—an irritation with the appearance of a sunburn.

Other common side effects include vomiting and fatigue. Such side effects are typical in radiation protocols used to treat brain tumors, but according to Dr. Hahn are generally not evident when radiation is used in the Half Body Irradiation protocol to treat lymphoma. This is due to the fact that the dosages are smaller and are given less frequently.

THERAPIES IN THE PIPELINE

Shortly after Bullet's diagnosis, a veterinarian recommended a certain alternative cancer treatment. I read the literature and asked Dr. Hoskins and Dr. Porzio to read it as well. After hearing their thoughts, I decided against this treatment.

Knowledge Is Power

by Dr. Philip J. Bergman

I'm happy to have this opportunity to be a part of a book that will help so many pets and the people that love them. To begin, you are very likely reading this because your pet has been diagnosed with cancer. That word can be a very frightening one, but we have dramatically improved the care of veterinary cancer patients over the last 20 to 30 years.

Information and education will empower you to make the best decisions for your pet. This information can come from a variety of sources, including Web sites and newsgroups on the Internet, via personal contacts and via your veterinarian. Information provided in this book will help you to find all of these resources.

The very best information can be obtained from a veterinary medical oncologist who will fully assess your pet and then give you the various diagnostic and treatment alternatives based on their knowledge of the rapidly advancing field of veterinary cancer treatment.

One of the most common questions that I'm asked by pet owners relates to what they can do at home for their pet diagnosed with cancer. First and foremost, love your pet no differently that you normally would. Remember, they don't know they have cancer and so they don't suffer the psychological implications of the diagnosis as we do.

Next, don't change too many things at home at once (e.g. diet, surroundings and daily routines). If you decide to make some changes, do so slowly, one thing at a time, so that your pet has a chance to adjust. The stress that develops from having to adjust to too many changes at once can actually make a dog sick. It can then become difficult to differentiate between the effects of a progression of the cancer vs. changes in the home.

In my work, I have developed a strong interest in immunology as it relates to the treatment and, potentially, the prevention of cancer in pets. These areas are so rapidly evolving that, in my opinion, immunotherapy will become a standardized treatment option for pets with cancer over the next 5 to 10 years, with the hope of actual licensed products for veterinary usage becoming available in the next 3 to 5 years.

Molecular pathology is another important field involved in the fight against canine cancer. My laboratory is at the cutting edge in the development of "prognostic marker panels" for dogs with mast cell tumors or lymphoma. These panels enable clinicians to provide superior prognostic information. Similar panels for other tumors (e.g., mammary) are currently in development.

In closing, my heart goes out to you, your family and, most importantly, your pet. What you and your pet are about to go through is a war, and it's a war worth fighting. With the help of a good team including you, your veterinarian, your veterinary oncologist and a great support team, your pet has the best chance for a good quality life.

Philip J. Bergman DVM, PhD, diplomate ACVIM (Oncology), head of the Donaldson-Atwood Cancer Clinic & Flaherty Comparative Oncology Laboratory (Animal Medical Center, New York, NY), Adjunct Associate Faculty Member at the Memorial Sloan-Kettering Cancer Center and President of the Veterinary Cancer Society.

The therapy that I turned down might turn out to be the "Magic Bullet" against canine lymphoma. My point is that because there is an almost endless list of treatments and supplements available, selectivity is necessary. Based on what? Based on research, test results, empirical data, advice from your canine cancer team members...and based on your own gut instincts.

Many new treatments are being developed to fight canine cancer. They are at various stages in the research and development process. Some are being studied in Petri dishes in laboratories at schools of veterinary medicine while others that are farther along in the process are being used to treat cancer-dogs in clinical trials.

All have the potential to become effective tools in the fight against canine cancer. They have yet to be tested for safety and consistency of results and then fine-tuned. In many cases, the therapy is known to be effective, but it has not yet been fine-tuned. Trials help to establish the big picture and then the details of precisely how a tool can be used most effectively.

When considering these unproven treatments for your dog, keep in mind that the further along the therapy is in the development process, the more confidence you can have that it will be an effective treatment.

CRYOSURGERY

This treatment type is most often used for tumors on the skin, eyelid and perianal area and for oral tumors. Liquid nitrogen or nitrous oxide is used to "freeze" the tumor. Tumor sites that should not be treated with cryosurgery include Osteosarcoma of long bones, Intranasal tumors, circumferential anus, large mast cell tumors and large, aggressive tumors.

Relative to traditional surgery, cryosurgery is a shorter procedure with less trauma to the dog, does not require anesthesia and is less costly. The downside is that there's no way to know whether or not "clear margins" have been achieved (whether or not all surrounding tissue containing cancer cells was treated).[1]

If your dog has a tumor and cryosurgery is suggested as a treatment, consult a veterinary oncologist before choosing this option. After cryosurgery, a biopsy can no longer be performed to determine if the tumor was benign or malignant and testing for clean margins is not possible.

HYPERTHERMIA

In a way, hyperthermia is the opposite of cryotherapy. The temperature of tumor cells is raised by ultrasound, microwaves or radiofrequency electrocautery. This treatment hasn't had positive results, but may someday play a role in the fight against cancer, in combination with radiation therapy or chemotherapy. Dr. J. Paul Woods writes, "Hyperthermia offers potential benefit to pets with recurrent, progressive, resistant cancer not amenable to standard therapies."[2]

PHOTODYNAMIC THERAPY (PDT)

Like cryotherapy and hyperthermia, this treatment exposes cancer cells to a stimulus in hopes that they will, as a result, become damaged (cytotoxicity) and die (necrosis). The goal of these treatment methods—and the goal of most tumor treatment—is to destroy tumor tissue but not the surrounding normal tissues.

In the case of Photodynamic Therapy, the stimulus is a three-way combination that includes a photosensitizer (IV or topically) to make the tissue more responsive to the treatment; a light source (usually laser) and oxygen that is required to complete the photochemical oxidative process.

PDT is in use in veterinary medicine, according to Dr. Dudley McCaw, DVM, diplomate ACVIM, for two types of canine cancer: Transitional cell carcinoma and canine oral squamous cell carcinoma. It's been approved for use in humans, in various countries, for lung, esophageal, bladder and gastric cancers.[3]

Studies show that there's a potential for PDT treatment to benefit cancer patients in the future. Much is still unknown about exactly how it works and how to make it work more efficiently.

IMMUNOTHERAPY

Studies are underway designed to explore the possibility of fighting and/or curing cancer through immunotherapy. This is a very complex and fascinating technology that is showing some initial signs of success.

Monoclonal antibody (mab) therapy, for example, has made inroads in the fight against cancer in recent years. In a process called Xenomouse technology, mice are stimulated to produce large amounts of antibodies—not just any antibodies, but the specific antibodies that are produced to fight a specific cancer cell in a specific species.

Monoclonal antibodies are therefore disease-specific and species-specific. This means that the mab for one type of canine cancer is different from the mab for another type of canine cancer (disease-specific) and the mab for a certain cancer in canines is different from the mab for that cancer in humans (species-specific).

Once produced, the antibodies are extracted and later delivered to the cancer patient intravenously. Mabs are called "targeted therapies" because they affect a very specific cancer cell and (unlike chemotherapy) do not harm healthy cells.

Two mab's (Rituxan and Zevalin) have been approved for use in fighting Non-Hodgkin's Lymphoma in humans. Another (Herceptin) combats breast cancer in humans. These are available and in common use. Joseph A. Impellizeri, DVM and residency-trained Medical Oncologist at Advanced Veterinary Care in Newburgh, NY says that because Rituxan was found to be ineffective in the canine, "It is unlikely that any of these newer targeted therapies used in people will be added to our armamentarium of therapeutics for our canine lymphoma patients."

The monoclonal antibody developed to fight canine lymphoma is called mab-231. Mab-231 was available shortly before Bullet's diagnosis. It was used, in most cases, not instead of chemotherapy but with it. I was interested to learn more about mab-231 and conducted a very thorough search for information about it. I contacted the laboratory that developed it and the distributor as well, but it was no longer available. The representatives I spoke to said that it has vanished, possibly due to a lack of demand.

Immunocytochemistry is another cutting-edge tool that is helpful not in treatment, but in the diagnosis and prognosis of canine lymphoma.

According to Dr. Impellizeri,

This modality [immunocytochemistry] allows oncologists to evaluate a canine lymphoma patient for B and T cell markers without needing to anesthetize and perform a surgical biopsy. A simple needle aspirate from the lymph node...is all it takes to learn which phenotype is expressed. I anticipate this will become a common diagnostic tool in the near future.

ANTIANGIOGENESIS THERAPY

Angio (blood or lymph vessel) genesis (birth) is the development of new blood vessels. Without the blood supply provided by a specific type of vessel, tumors are unable to grow. *Anti* angiogenesis therapy introduces substances that have been found to selectively inhibit the generation of these new vessels, thereby cutting off the blood supply to tumors and, as it were, starving them to death.

Chand Khanna DVM, PhD, diplomate ACVIM (oncology), President of the Animal Cancer Institute and Chairman of the Perseus Foundation, is involved in research using antiangiogenic agents. Dr. Khanna explains this treatment as follows:

Agents that inhibit new blood vessel formation or specifically target tumor-associated blood vessels represent a novel, potentially effective and non-toxic treatment for cancer. It is likely that these agents will provide the next major break-through in the management of pet animals and people with cancer...in combination with surgery, radiation therapy and chemotherapy.[4]

One antiangiogenesis success story involves a dog named Navy. As of July 2002, Navy had maintained a 16-month remission from lymphoma due to this treatment. This "cure" has not been repeated successfully but has instigated new research in the field in both veterinary and human oncology. [5]

VACCINE THERAPY

There is a great deal of ongoing research in the area of vaccine therapy for canine malignant melanoma. Dr. Bergman, who is involved in this research, states:

Canine malignant melanoma (CMM) is an aggressive cancer that commonly spreads and is resistant to standardized therapies. Novel therapies are desperately needed for this extremely malignant tumor. At present, standardized therapies generally translates to median survival times (MST) of 3 to 6 months for dogs with advanced CMM. However, the MST for dogs with advanced CMM treated with surgery or radiation followed by DNA vaccine is approaching 2 years.

CLINICAL TRIALS

New clinical trials in veterinary oncology are announced on an ongoing basis. Most aim to compare the success rate of an accepted protocol with its success rate when given over an abbreviated or extended time period, in different amounts, dosages, titrations, combinations and/or on a different schedule. There are also clinical trials that are designed to test the efficacy of a new type of cancer treatment or one that's been newly revised.

Through trials, cancer treatment has been improved over the years. Side effects have been minimalized and survival rates have improved. Some day, probably as the result of a clinical trial, a treatment that has a high success rate with minimal drawbacks will be discovered.

The announcement of a clinical trial states that the trial is in progress, explains the procedure and specifies the requirements for enrollment. Most trials have strict requirements for enrollment. Some specify that only dogs who have not undergone chemotherapy and/or radiation therapy are candidates, or are within a certain age range. Some are open only to dogs who are in a first remission; others only to dogs who have relapsed (have come out of remission) several times.

During a clinical trial, participants (dogs with cancer) are monitored closely to document side effects, general health and, of course, survival time. In some trials, particularly those using an experimental drug, funding is available to help caretakers manage the costs. Participants may be required to forgo other treatments that have documented success or to grant permission for an autopsy to be performed on the dog if he dies during the trial.

A clinical trial may reveal a new, successful treatment that will not only help your dog but also many other dogs—and, eventually, people—with cancer. Conversely, a clinical trial may prove to be less effective than traditional treatments. When no traditional treatment with a high success rate is available, however, or if budgetary constraints preclude other treatment, enrollment in a clinical trial is a very attractive option.

To learn out about clinical trials in which your dog might be a candidate, you might start by asking your veterinarian or veterinary oncologist about trials in which he is participating or to which he has access. If you discover a trial appropriate for your dog, you can return to your veterinarian to ask if he can become a participant in the trial.

Many clinical trials are conducted at schools of veterinary medicine. Refer to the list on page 22 to research these. Trials are also conducted at clinical referral practices. These are veterinary practices that participate in networks such as the Animal Cancer Network or the Gulf Coast Network. According to Dr. Hahn, the Gulf Coast Network includes four regional practices and a network of over 20 primary care practices. Each of these 24

CLINICAL TRIAL ANNOUNCEMENT

Antiangiogenic therapy for dogs with any measurable cancer

Status: Open
Eligibility:

- measurable disease defined by examination, radiographs or ultrasound

- no cytotoxic therapy within 3 weeks of trial initiation

- prednisone or NSAID therapy permitted if introduced at least 3 weeks before trial initiation

- No previous antiangiogenic therapy

Trial Support: Study patients receive Thrombospondin -I peptide at no charge. Medical examinations and diagnostic tests needed to measure response are the responsibility of the owner. All cases must be evaluated and treated through the Animal Cancer Institute primary clinic site at Friendship Hospital for Animals, Washington DC. Diagnostic tests may be performed at any veterinary hospital within 10 days of initiation of study

See all participating sites for this clinical trial

Reprinted by permission of the Animal Cancer Institute

practices can include clients (caretakers) and patients (dogs with cancer) in any clinical trial being conducted under the umbrella of the Gulf Coast Network.

Many large veterinary hospitals with specialty services participate in trials as well. Contact those in your area to inquire whether there are clinical trials in progress in which your dog might be a participant.

Organizations such as the Animal Cancer Institute and the Veterinary Cancer Society provide information about clinical trials as well.

References

1 *Small Animal Clinical Oncology,* editors Stephen J. Withrow, DVM, diplomate ACVIM (oncology) and E. Gregory MacEwen, VMD, diplomate ACVIM (oncology and internal medicine). W.B. Saunders Company, 2001, p.82.

2 *Veterinary Oncology Secrets,* editor Robert C. Rosenthal, DVM, PhD. Hanley & Belfus, Inc, 2001, p.87.

3 ibid, p.90.

4 "Targeting the blood supply of cancer," by Chand Khanna DVM, PhD, Dipl ACVIM (Oncology), 2002. [www. TheAnimalCancerInstitute.com]

5 "Dog's Complete Cancer Cure Opens New Doors In Research," by Erin Kirk. *USA Today,* July 25, 2002.

CHEMOTHERAPY

*C*ancer may be the "C word" that makes us cringe most, but Chemotherapy is at least a close runner up. Chemotherapy is used to treat various types of cancer in dogs, including lymphoma, acute lymphoid leukemia, chronic lymphocytic leukemia, acute and chronic myelogenous leukemia, multiple myeloma, systemic mast cell tumors, soft-tissue sarcomas, osteosarcoma and carcinomas.[1]

Chemotherapy protocols designed for dogs are less rigorous than are those designed for humans. While many people are willing to undergo extreme, potentially life-threatening treatment in order to have a chance at beating cancer, most pet caretakers are not willing to see their dogs die or become severely ill from treatment. A chemotherapy protocol that is highly toxic can be expected to fall out of favor, even if it has also been found to be highly successful. Dr. Hahn explains,

> *Dogs tend to tolerate chemotherapy better than people do. This is because veterinarians rarely administer maximum dosages—those that would be most aggressive against cancer but would also guarantee severe side effects. Rather, we give dosages that will make only about 10 percent of pets have side effects. Survival times and remission times reported are based upon these "kinder, gentler" dosages. Consult with your veterinary team about your goals and expectations of chemotherapy when your pet is treated.*

EARLY DETECTION OF CANCER OR OF RELAPSE
by Dr. Rodney Page

Early detection is key to the successful treatment of canine cancer. All dog owners should watch for the early signs of cancer that are listed in the "Ten Common Signs of Cancer in Small Animals" and report any and all findings to their veterinarian.

These signs may also indicate that a dog in remission with cancer has relapsed or developed new cancer sites. In many instances, the need for a second remission does not mean that treatment can no longer provide additional quality time.

I recommend that all dog owners examine their dogs monthly according to the following list. Owners of dogs that have been diagnosed with cancer should conduct the same examination weekly.

The Ten Common Signs of Cancer in Small Animals

▶ Abnormal swellings that persist or continue to grow

▶ Sores that do not heal

▶ Weight loss

▶ Loss of appetite

▶ Bleeding or discharge from any body opening

▶ Offensive odor

▶ Difficulty eating or swallowing

▶ Hesitation to exercise or loss of stamina

▶ Persistent lameness or stiffness

▶ Difficulty breathing, urinating or defecating

1. Feel your dog's lymph node regions. See page 13 for a map of the locations of the major lymph nodes on a dog or ask your veterinarian to show you where the nodes are on your dog. Make a note of the size of each node—a mental note and also a notation in your log book for later reference.

2. Feel the mammary glands on female dogs to detect any changes.

3. Go over the skin of your dog's entire body. Make "dermal maps" of any existing lumps and bumps. This will later help you determine how quickly a benign skin bump may be changing.

4. Try to examine the inside of your dog's mouth. This is sometimes challenging but is often easier than expected, depending on the dog's disposition.

5. Annual blood and urine tests are adequate unless there are any abnormalities. Then, schedule rechecks every 4 to 6 months to follow those abnormal results.

6. Twice a year, if possible, your dog should have chest X-rays and abdominal ultrasound, particularly in breeds that are predisposed to splenic hemangiosarcoma (Golden Retrievers and German Shepherd dogs). Although this may sound excessive, remember that dogs age much faster than do humans. An annual visit to the veterinarian is simply not sufficient to protect a geriatric dog.

Rodney Page, DVM, diplomate ACVIM (Internal Medicine, Oncology) is a professor and the director of the Sprecher Institute for Comparative Cancer Research at the College of Veterinary Medicine, Cornell University.

Lymphoma is said to be the most aggressive form of canine cancer. Most experts—including most holistic veterinarians who are generally opposed to the use of chemotherapy for treating cancer—agree that dogs diagnosed with lymphoma have a life expectancy of only a few weeks without chemotherapy.

Lymphoma is also said to be highly treatable. According to Susan M. Cotter DVM, diplomate ACVIM (Internal Medicine/Oncology), Tufts University School of Veterinary Medicine, with chemotherapy, "Dogs with lymphoma have an average survival of around a year past diagnosis with a good quality of life."

GET A MOVE ON!

It's best not to deliberate the point too long— get started ASAP and you can iron out the fine points, even switch oncologists or treatment plans, later. Why the urgency? In most cancers, the sooner you begin, the better the prognosis. Cancer can also grow or spread rapidly if left untreated.

In about 80 percent of canine lymphoma cases that are treated with chemotherapy, remission is achieved within the first few treatments—often with a single treatment. Without chemotherapy, lymphoma and other cancers grow increasingly "stronger" and more widespread and thus more difficult to treat.

Once cancer cells migrate into the bloodstream and form a new tumor in a different part of the body, the cancer is said to have "metastasized." Once metastasis has occurred, the disease will continue to progress. At this point, the prognosis worsens considerably.

According to Dr. Cotter, Lymphoma and leukemia are considered to be systemic from the beginning.

> Like most cancers, these cancers begin as a single cell. However, because these cells are abnormal variants of blood cells, and can thus easily travel through the blood or lymphatic system, the diseases seem to start in many places or in the lymph nodes all at once.

Until remission is achieved, active cancer cells are busily damaging the body's vital organs including the kidney, spleen, lungs and liver. Many of the cancer-fighting agents used in chemotherapy can themselves cause damage to these organs and to the heart. Once the damage is done, the dog, caretaker and veterinarian are left with not only the cancer to combat, but organ damage or dysfunction as well.

Dr. Cotter says, "A dog that is asymptomatic (i.e., only has enlarged lymph nodes) has a better chance of remission than a dog that has other symptomology related to cancer." The healthier the organs are at the start of chemotherapy, the better able your dog will be to tolerate the internal maelstrom that is created by chemotherapy.

According to Dr. Ruslander, in the case of lymphoma, the stage of the disease does not necessarily determine the potential success of treatment "...unless there's stage V extranodal or bone marrow involvement."

Dr. Porzio agrees, adding that the outcome of chemotherapy treatment for lymphoma appears to be the same regardless of when it begins, so long as there's no organ involvement (no signs that cancer cells are present in an organ); that the dog is asymptomatic other than enlarged lymph nodes and that at the time cancer treatment begins, the dog has not been previously treated with prednisone alone.

Drugs in the corticosteroid family (such as prednisone), when given alone, can induce a phenomenon called "multidrug resistance."

> *Prednisone used as a single agent may induce drug resistance...If an owner opts to try prednisone alone first and asks for combination therapy later, the results may not be as good as usually expected.*[2]

For dogs with lymphoma in chemotherapy, remission is usually achieved quickly in 80 to 90 percent of cases. The duration of the remission, however, varies greatly but generally lasts between 3 and 18 months.

With a diagnosis of cancer, we'd all prefer to hear "early stage," but whenever the disease is discovered is the time that you begin. Since it isn't possible to go back in time and discover it at an earlier stage, do what you can now. According to the pathologist's report on Bullet's biopsy, the lymphoma was "late stage." Nonetheless, the first chemotherapy treatment achieved a remission that has lasted nearly four years.

CHEMOTHERAPY SIMPLIFIED

Briefly, chemotherapy is the application of one or more "agents" designed to kill cancer cells or at least hinder their ability to multiply and damage healthy cells. Some agents are administered intravenously, others are injected subcutaneously and others are given in pill form, orally.

No one of these agents reliably "cures" cancer. Even though there *is* no "Magic Bullet" (except for the one snoozing in my living room), each chemotherapy agent is effective to some degree,

ABOUT PROTOCOLS

A protocol is an attack plan of sorts. It specifies the agents (drugs) that will be given, the dosages and the schedule by which they will be given, week by week, from beginning to end. The choice of a protocol is a strategic decision, similar to deciding whether to deploy the marines, the air force or the navy to attack an enemy.

There are two very general types of protocols: single agent protocols, which use one agent repeatedly until the patient comes out of remission, and combination protocols. The combination protocols are favored.

Each chemotherapy agent attacks cancer in a different way (i.e., at a different stage during the replication of the cancer cell). Agents are rotated according to a schedule in an attempt to "hit" the cancer with one, then another, then another, hoping for a better shot at killing as many cancer cells as possible (or at least giving them a TKO or a concussion).

Each protocol is unique insofar as which agents it includes, in what order and on what schedule. Many protocol names are composed of the first letters of the agents employed. Because there's a limited number of agents available, similarities between

protocol names, such as CHOP, COP, CLOP and MOPP are common. Most include Prednisone, thus the final "P."

When remission is achieved, this does not mean that chemotherapy ends. In most cases, the cancer will return quickly if treatment is stopped before the end of the protocol. Just as it's known that a full course of antibiotics should be taken even if the patient is feeling better, so the entire chemotherapy protocol should be completed.

The duration of a protocol is determined by studies conducted to find the point of diminishing returns. This is the point beyond which the average survival of dogs tested does not increase if chemotherapy treatments continue.

If a dog comes out of remission, an attempt is made to acquire a second remission. This time around, it's called "second line" chemotherapy.

If the dog comes out of remission after the protocol is completed, the same protocol may be used again. If, however, remission is achieved and the dog relapses before completing the chemotherapy protocol, then most likely the cancer has become resistant to the drugs used to obtain

the first remission and they are not used again—they have already failed. A new drug or combination of drugs is employed.

In the case of canine lymphoma, there's an 80 percent success rate for achieving a first remission and a 40 percent success rate in achieving a second one (approximations). In general, a second remission may last about half the length of time as the first and generally, each subsequent remission lasts a shorter period of time. Some dogs have been in and out of remission five times or more.

"Chemotherapy is not an exact science." Dr. Porzio said this many times during Bullet's treatment. If your dog reacts badly to one of the agents in your protocol, you and your oncologist can agree to customize the protocol for your dog. You might, for example, give him a smaller dose of the offending agent when it appears in the schedule. Or you may decide to skip it entirely and replace it with a different agent.

Any deviation from a protocol should be decided on only under the expert consultation of your dog's medical team, most importantly his veterinary oncologist.

alone or in combination with other agents. Much of the research done involves studying the agents in different combinations and permutations to determine which grouping, in what dosages and on what time schedule has the best results. These various treatment plans are called "protocols" (see "About Protocols," page 49).

The development of a new protocol often begins at a veterinary school where veterinary oncologists select a new combination of agents, a new treatment schedule and/or a variation of dosages. Before being accepted as a viable treatment, a new protocol is evaluated in a clinical trial. Clinical trials for pets with cancer are underway at most veterinary colleges and oncology specialty practices (see "Clinical Trials," page 42).

CHEMOTHERAPY AGENTS

Bullet's chemotherapy protocol, VELCAP-L (the L stands for long), had an excellent success rate but was very long, costly and was also cardiotoxic (damaging to the heart). Gerald S. Post, DVM, diplomate ACVIM (oncology), founder and president of the Animal Cancer Foundation, examined Bullet and said that the VELCAP-L protocol had fallen out of favor in the three years since Bullet's

treatment due to its cardiotoxicity. Dr. Cotter explains the trend toward shorter protocols:

Most dogs—particularly those with B-cell lymphoma as opposed to T-cell—don't require 18 months of chemotherapy. We now routinely test the biopsy specimen at the time of the original diagnosis to determine which type of lymphoma is present.

Doxorubicin is one of the most powerful chemotherapy agents available. It's included in most chemotherapy protocols for canine (and human) lymphoma, hemangiosarcoma, osteosarcoma and other cancers. This agent is also cardiotoxic and may eventually cause congestive heart failure. Recommendations are issued for a lifetime maximum amount of Doxorubicin but Dr. Impellizeri explains that there are exceptions to this generalization as follows:

Despite Doxorubicin's known cardiotoxicity, it still may be administered past the maximum recommended dose. This is contingent, of course, on no evidence of any cardiac pathology identified up until that point. Sometimes Doxorubicin is the only drug that is effective at holding an animal's lymphoma in remission. In addition, the amount of time that the drug is administered over can contribute to this cardiotoxicity with unpublished research by my mentor indicating that the longer the period of time over which the drug is administered, the lower the chance of cardiotoxicity.

Some dogs tolerate Doxorubicin with no ill effects and others become quite ill. If signs of early heart disease are detected, even if the lifetime maximum amount has not been given, this drug will not ever again be used on that dog.

A Delicate Procedure

Some chemotherapy agents that are administered intravenously can be absorbed through the skin. A catheter is inserted into the dog's vein and the medicine is delivered via the catheter to ensure that the fluid does not contact the dog's body tissue outside of the vein. The chemotherapy agent is flushed through the catheter into the vein while the dog is held still.

Members of a veterinary team administering intravenous (IV) chemotherapy wear latex gloves to ensure that the agent does not contact their skin. Chemotherapy agents are expelled from the dog's body through urine, feces or excreta. Some are still "active" after being expelled and will, on contact, enter a person's bloodstream. For this reason, vigorous cleanup wearing latex gloves is necessary so that other dogs, cats and/or people do not make contact with the still-active chemical.

Most treatments take less than an hour, but the duration depends on which agent is being administered and also on how cooperative the dog is on that day. The duration also varies depending on the size of the dog. The larger the dog, the greater the volume of chemotherapy agents given and thus the longer the duration of treatment.

Bullet's Chemo Experience

During Bullet's first chemotherapy sessions, he was decidedly not the model patient. He cried, he squirmed, he growled. Once he even nipped Rod (the fellow whose job it was to get Bullet to stay still). However, after the first few treatments, Bullet became a favorite patient. In fact, Dr. Porzio often emerged from a treatment saying that Bullet had been "an angel." He would lie still, quietly and comfortably and giving kisses to the workers holding him still. Most dogs become less afraid of and more agreeable to treatment in a short time.

At Bullet's first treatment, Dr. Porzio came out to tell me that he was having difficulty finding a vein in which to insert a catheter, through which the chemotherapy agent would be delivered. When I returned after 40 minutes, Bullet emerged with a shaved square on each of his four limbs.

For the following year, I asked Dr. Porzio to continue to use the vein in Bullet's left rear left leg, reshaving the same patch when necessary and allowing the fur to grow in over the other patches. After the first year of chemotherapy, I asked Dr. Porzio to switch to the right rear and give the left rear vein a rest. Eventually, a vein used repeatedly may collapse or become irritated and I feared that we were pushing our luck.

As any veterinarian who's worked on Bullet will attest, I am strongly against Bullet's fur being shaved unnecessarily. I thought that Dr. Goldstein expressed this sentiment beautifully when he told me that it's important to preserve the beauty and natural integrity of the animal whenever possible.

An ultrasound examination of Bullet's heart was performed before each treatment with the agent Doxorubicin. Although no signs of early heart disease were detected, Bullet consistently became very ill from this agent and we discontinued its use long before his lifetime maximum quantity was reached.

Some veterinarians prefer to treat a fasted dog. If your oncologist has no objections, encourage your dog to drink water before intravenous chemotherapy treatments. This will dilate his veins and make the insertion of the catheter simpler for the doctor and less traumatic for your dog.

References

1 *Manual of Small Animal Internal Medicine*, by Richard W. Nelson, DVM and C. Guillermo Couto, DVM. Mosby, 1999, pp.711-715.

2 *Veterinary Oncology Secrets*, editor Robert C. Rosenthal, DVM, PhD. Hanley & Belfus, Inc, 2001, p.183-4.

SIDE EFFECTS

Every prescription drug has a set of related side effects. Some are common and others occurred only in a small percentage of the test population. Likewise, each chemotherapy agent has a set of reactions that were experienced by a certain percentage of clinical trial participants.

Still, these are only statistics. Some dogs are overly sensitive to all of the agents and become ill from each treatment. Others suffer side effects only to particular agents. Still others seem immune to all side effects from any agent and withstand every treatment without any sign of illness.

Your dog may not have typical reactions to chemotherapy treatments. He may have reactions not included in the list of common side effects.

When serious side effects do occur, dosages are decreased in subsequent treatments and, more often than not, the dog tolerates the lower dose. Most dogs will react more or less consistently to each chemotherapy agent. After your dog's first treatment with each agent, you'll be prepared for his reaction the next time this agent is given.

If your dog has an adverse reaction to a chemotherapy treatment, don't hesitate to inform your veterinarian or oncologist right away. He might be able to provide medication, or there might be something you can do at home to stop the reaction. He might say to bring your pet into the clinic right away or not to worry because the reaction is normal and is not dangerous.

KEEP YOUR DOG HEALTHY DURING CHEMOTHERAPY
by Dr. Kevin A. Hahn

Your dog has cancer and you feel helpless. His body is turning against itself and your veterinary oncologist has said that nothing can be done to cure your dog but chemotherapy may delay the inevitable.

Are you helpless? No! There are measures that you and your veterinary team can take to minimize chemotherapy side effects and allow your dog to enjoy a longer, better quality life.

Chemotherapy side effects occur because the agents are designed to kill rapidly growing cells. The vast majority of cells killed are cancer cells. However, bone marrow and cells of the intestinal lining also grow rapidly and are killed by chemotherapy as innocent bystanders.

Bone marrow and the intestine produce a certain percentage of new cells every day and those cells are "reserved" to be used by the body 1 to 3 days later. For this reason, most complications from chemotherapy occur 1 to 3 days after treatment.

▸ **Be Observant:** Be sure to report all chemotherapy side effects to your veterinarian. If treatment is needed, it should begin as early as possible in order to get the best result.

▸ **Check for Fever:** If your dog seems tired, lethargic or weak, don't rely on body warmth, a wet or dry nose or panting—take his rectal temperature. Fever may be caused by low white blood cell count (neutropenia) or by the death of tumor cells (non-infectious inflammation) and may be treated with intravenous fluids or antibiotics. Normal temperature in a dog ranges from 100.0 to 103.5 degrees Fahrenheit.

▸ **Feed Wisely:** There's no universally accepted "good diet" for pets on chemotherapy. A well-balanced diet that is easy to digest (requiring less work from the intestine), easily absorbed (generating less stool, hence less diarrhea) and high in calories (to avoid weight loss and protein loss) is best.

The recommended diet is low in carbohydrates, high in the non-inflammatory fats (Omega N-3 fatty acids or fish oils) and provides good quality protein (from egg or poultry products). Consult with your veterinary team about the commercial, prescription or homemade diet that's right for your pet's body condition, breed and diagnosis.

Alternative treatments and immune stimulants may be helpful, but always consult with your veterinarian and provide a list of all supplements at each visit. Some may worsen side effects of chemotherapy or interfere with treatment.

▸ **Promote Wellness:** Some serious complications can arise long after the completion of chemotherapy. Because these delayed problems may occur months to years after treatment and because they often go unnoticed, regular veterinary examinations are warranted. Other health-care measures, including heartworm prevention and flea control, are still necessary.

The essential rule for good home care is "when in doubt, check it out." Tell your veterinary team about every concern that you have.

Kevin A. Hahn, DVM, PhD, diplomate ACVIM (Oncology), PhD, practicing in Houston and San Antonio, Texas.

Now that you have a whole "team" of experts contributing to your dog's well-being, you'll have to decide which team member or members to call on for assistance when a problem arises. Call one or all—in time, you'll learn who is most accessible and who has the best solutions. Don't forget to make a notation in your log with all of the details of the episode, including what it was that finally helped.

The following section is an overview of common side effects, each followed by some of the available remedies. This is not by any means a comprehensive list. For additional information, see "Recommended Reading," page 107.

VOMITING AND NAUSEA

- Clean up! The vomitus may contain toxic chemicals that were not absorbed into your dog's system, so clean up as best you can and always wear protective gloves. Outdoors, dissipate the vomitus by pouring water over it so that other animals don't lick it up. Indoors, pick up what you can and then use water or a pet stain cleanser to remove the rest.

- Watch for signs of dehydration. To test, pick up the skin on the scruff of your dog's neck, where a pup's mother (that is, his genetic mother) would grab on to carry the pup. Then let go. If the skin doesn't fall down flat on your dog's neck within a few seconds, he may be dehydrated and you should call your veterinarian. Call your veterinarian if there is any blood in the vomitus, if vomiting persists for more than two days or if your dog vomits more than three times in a 24-hour period.

- Dr. Cotter says that antiemetics can prevent vomiting in dogs undergoing chemotherapy. If your dog vomits after a treatment, report this to your oncologist. Before the next treatment that includes the offending agent, he can pre-treat your dog with antiemetics.

    Prescription (Rx): Your veterinarian may prescribe an antinausea (antiemetic) drug such as Reglan® or one of the more potent (and also more expensive) antiemetic drugs such as Zofran® or Anzemet®.

    Over The Counter (OTC): PeptoBismol® (check with your veterinarian first), particularly after chemotherapy agent doxorubicin is given. Pepcid AC® (check with your veterinarian first)

    Other: Ginger is a good natural remedy for nausea L-Glutamine: If your dog takes this regularly, double the amount while vomiting persists. (Do not give your dog L-Glutamine if he has epilepsy or is taking anti-seizure medication.)

    Nux Vomica 6C

DIARRHEA

▸ Again, clean up!

▸ Watch for mucous (a loose stool that glistens and/or hangs before falling to the ground; a liquid stool that's shiny with consistency of uncooked egg white). If you suspect there is mucous in your dog's stools, report this to your veterinarian.

▸ Projectile diarrhea: This is a shocking occurrence for the caretaker and, I can only surmise, for the dog. Try to stay out of the spray zone—otherwise, treat the same as ordinary diarrhea.

Rx: Metronidozole: To decrease inflammation.

OTC: PeptoBismol; Imodium®; Lomotil. Check with your veterinarian before giving these remedies.

Other: Do not give vitamin C or CoQ10.

Temporarily decrease oil (fatty acids) in food.

L-Glutamine: *Do not give L-Glutamine if your dog has epilepsy or is taking antiseizure medication.

Acidophilus and bifidus: As chewable tablets or in organic yogurt.

Potato, brown rice, sweet potato, pumpkin: Only until the diarrhea stops.

Pectin: Mix a teaspoon of powdered pectin with filtered water in a needle-less syringe and empty it slowly into your dog's mouth.

High-fiber bran cereal: Sprinkled it onto a meal or mix with water as above.

BLOODY DIARRHEA

▸ The lining of a dog's intestines can be damaged by chemotherapy agents. If you see blood in your dog's stool, notify your veterinary oncologist immediately and make a note in your log. If bleeding occurs in the intestines, the stool may appear black rather than red because of the distance between the source and the exit point.

If the bleeding doesn't stop within two days (or sooner if severe), an examination will be necessary.

Remedies: Same as those listed for diarrhea.

NOT EATING

▸ Loss of appetite can indicate the presence of infection. Check your dog's temperature and alert your veterinarian if it is above 103 degrees Fahrenheit.

▸ Don't panic, but do try anything and everything. Start with foods that are healthy and cancer-conscious, but resort to anything. The longer he doesn't eat, the less inclined he will be to start eating—in other words, "not eating" can become habitual.

▸ Feed Frozen. Heating food to combat nausea is often recommended but in my experience has not been effective. I've had great success with frozen or semi-frozen food (see "Feeding Frozen," page 68).

Rx: Antiemetics may be prescribed since loss of appetite may be due to nausea.

OTC: Pepcid AC, Rescue Remedy

Other: Frozen fish, cottage cheese, ginger, garlic

"FLAT OUT"

When a dog is nonresponsive, not eating and hardly moving, I call this condition "flat out." Dr. Ruslander advises that this condition is important because,

> This could represent neutropenia [low neutrophil count—neutrophils are a type of WBC] or sepsis [high levels of toxin in the blood], which is the most concerning acute side effect that veterinary oncologists worry about. If the dog is febrile (has a temperature above 103 degrees F.), this is a life-threatening emergency.

Dr. Cotter says that when a dog is febrile, bactericidal antibiotics such as a combination of gentamicin and cephalothin or fluoroquinolones are given intravenously until the neutrophil count rises. In most cases, this occurs within 2 to 3 days.

Your veterinarian will check your dog's white blood cell count and neutrophil level.

Check your dog's temperature.

Get him to eat! Try anything and everything. Appetite enhancers are generally not effective in dogs.

Rescue Remedy, Vitamin B-12

DIFFICULTY BREATHING

Some dogs have allergic reactions to certain chemotherapy agents in the form of respiratory distress. This may manifest as rasping, wheezing or reverse sneezing. Notify your oncologist or your veterinarian right away—anaphylactic shock is possible and can be fatal. If the cause is a sensitivity to a particular chemotherapy agent, the dosage of the agent may be decreased. If the symptoms are caused by an allergic reaction, use of the agent is discontinued entirely.

Inform your veterinarian immediately

Rx: Clavamox, one of the newer "designer" antibiotics, controlled this reaction very effectively for Bullet. Dr. Cotter says that antibiotics will help resolve this condition if it's caused by a respiratory infection such as pneumonia.

SWELLING

This may signal an allergic reaction to a chemotherapy agent or to the long-term use of prednisone. Swelling may also be caused by edema due to a tumor or by heart failure.

Inform your veterinarian immediately

HAIR LOSS

Dogs don't typically lose their hair during chemotherapy as do humans (with few exceptions, including poodles and other dogs that have "hair" rather than "fur" and some terriers). This is because hair growth for most dogs is seasonal, not continual. It is common, however, for dogs to lose their whiskers early on and to experience some hair loss if the chemotherapy continues for more than a few months.

Any fur clipped or shaved during chemotherapy will grow back, but only over a long period of time. Bullet's team members are aware of my opposition to any unnecessary shaving or clipping and go out of their way to oblige me.

Brush well to remove loose hair/fur
Nettles (dry herb flakes, crumbled on food)
Silica 500 supplement (health food store)

LOW WHITE BLOOD CELL COUNT

A CBC (Complete Blood Count) will be done regularly while your dog is in chemotherapy. A low neutrophil (one type of white blood cell) count may prompt your oncologist to suspend chemotherapy temporarily.

Rx: Antibiotics
Neupogen® (Filgrastim) may be prescribed to increase the number of neutrophils in the blood.

Other: Cancer-dog caretakers have reported that adding rinsed light red kidney beans to their dog's food between chemotherapy treatments helps to keep the white blood cell count from dropping.

ANEMIA

Although anemia (insufficient red blood cell count) is not a typical chemotherapy side effect, many dogs in cancer treatment become mildly anemic as a reaction to the immunosuppressive nature of chemotherapy. However, if the cancer has infiltrated the bone marrow and is not in remission, the red cells, white cells and platelets all become insufficient. The prognosis in this situation is very poor.

Rx: Procrit® is often prescribed
Aranesp® (darbepoetin alfa) treats anemia caused by chemotherapy

DON'T PANIC!

If your dog doesn't tolerate chemotherapy, you and your veterinary oncologist will probably agree to postpone treatment until the dog has recovered from the side effects. Treat the symptoms, make your dog as comfortable as possible and hope for a turnaround. Make use of your team members and pay attention to your own instincts, based on your intimate knowledge of your dog.

There are several possible courses of action that may be taken following severe side effects:

▸ Continue treatment according to protocol in hopes that your dog will better tolerate subsequent treatments.

▸ Continue treatment with revisions to the protocol, including amounts and types of agents used and/or the scheduling of treatments. If there is one specific chemotherapy agent that causes severe side effects in your dog, that agent can be omitted from the protocol and replaced with another or the dosage of the agent can be reduced in future treatments.

▸ Stop current treatment and initiate a different treatment modality, such as a standard but less widely used treatment for the dog's condition, an alternative therapy or a therapy that is in clinical trials.

▸ Stop treatment and provide palliative care.

If your dog doesn't respond to treatment as hoped and remission is not achieved, your veterinary oncologist may employ other agents or perhaps, depending on the type and location of the cancer, other therapies in an attempt to induce remission. Ultimately, if this fails, he will probably provide you with a new prognosis and a recommendation for palliative care.

At this point, you might make the decision to stop fighting and focus instead on maximizing your dog's quality of life. Remember that many dogs outlive their prognoses.

But, if you're not ready to give up the fight, there are still a few options that you can explore. Clinical trials, for example, often seek out dogs that have been resistant to standard therapies. Your holistic veterinarian can provide a selection of alternative therapies to choose from and you can also explore the library and the Internet for new approaches.

BULLET'S SIDE EFFECTS

For Bullet, chemotherapy began with a treatment of Doxorubicin. He showed no reaction at all except that he threw up lots of clear fluid once, a day later. I remember vividly because I was in the middle of a phone consult with Tina Aiken, a holistic veterinarian at Dr. Marty Goldstein's office who has been immensely helpful throughout. Bullet had a second Doxorubicin treatment a week later and this time he became extremely ill.

CHEMOTHERAPY AGENTS AND THEIR SIDE EFFECTS [1]

GENERIC NAME	BRAND NAME (®)	CLEARED VIA	CLEARANCE TIME	HOW GIVEN	SIDE EFFECTS
actinomycin-D	Cosmegen	Urine, Feces	7 days	IV	Vessels, Marrow, GI
doxorubicin	Adriamycin	Feces	7 days	IV infusion	Marrow, GI, Heart, Anaphylaxis
asparaginase	Elspar			IM or Subq	Allergy, Marrow
azathiope	Imuran	Urine	8 hours	Pill	Marrow, GI
carmustine	BCNU	Urine	4 days	IV	Marrow, Lungs, GI, Kidney
carboplatin	Paraplatin	Urine	1 day	IV infusion	Marrow, GI, Allergy
lomustine	CCNU	Degradation	1 day	Pill, IV	GI, Marrow, Lungs, Liver
chlorambucil	Leukeran	Urine	1 day	Pill	Marrow, GI
cisplatin	Platinol	Urine	1 day	IV, IV infusion	Kidney, GI, Marrow
cyclophosphamide	Cytoxan	Urine	72 hours	Pill, IV	Marrow, Kidney, GI
cytosine arabinoside	Cytosar-U	Urine	1 day	IV	Marrow, GI
etoposide/VP-16	VePesid	Urine	1 day	Pill, IV	Marrow, GI
melphalan	Alkeran	Urine	7 days	Pill, IV	Marrow
methotrexate	Trexsol	Urine	1 day	Pill, IV	GI, Marrow
mitoxantrone	Novantrone	Urine, Feces	7 days	IV infusion	GI, Marrow
paclitaxel	Taxol	Feces	5 days	IV	Marrow, GI, Anaphylaxis
prednisone				Pill	Weakness, Panting, Marrow, Cushings
vinblastine	Velban	Urine	72 hours	IV	Vessels, Marrow, GI
vincristine	Oncovin	Urine, Feces	7 days	IV	Vessles, Nerves, Marrow, GI

Bullet didn't eat for nearly two weeks. He was "flat out" 24/7, sometimes crying quietly. He needed my help to go outside to pee. There was blood in his stool and he was vomiting. I wondered if I was being unkind by keeping him alive.

Once, upon seeing Bullet's condition, a friend said, "You know, many people whose pets have cancer feel that euthanasia's a kinder option than treatment." Her message was clear and indeed I did question my decision to keep going then (and many other times when Bullet became ill), but in each case I decided "not yet." I had no way of knowing that Bullet would survive the episode. If he had not, would my decision have been the wrong one? Perhaps in retrospect it would have been, but in the absence of a crystal ball, I simply had to trust my instincts.

Bullet and I weathered a number of seemingly hopeless setbacks. With each new setback, I knew that this time could turn out to be the one that Bullet would not survive but I stored that understanding in the back of my mind and continued to believe, each time, that he would recover and simply went about taking care of him the best I could.

As for side effects, Bullet never once came out of the clinic after a chemotherapy treatment ill. I always waited for him because my schedule allowed it and because I wanted to avoid making Bullet wait in a cage, since he has a history of being cage-protective. At the end of every treatment, Bullet came trotting happily out of the treatment room. When Bullet suffered side effects, the symptoms usually appeared 5 to 10 days after a chemotherapy treatment. Many cancer-dog caretakers report that the onset of side effects often takes place 3 days to a week after treatment.

The first time Bullet had what I call a "flat out" reaction, he was practically motionless, lying on his side for nearly two weeks. He would get up only if I first lifted him to a half-standing position and he would not eat. He looked deflated. I thought that it would be a miracle if he pulled through.

Whenever Bullet had a flat out day during his protocol, Dr. Porzio or Dr. Hoskins would first ensure that he did not have a fever, that his white blood cell count (WBC) was adequate and that he was not dehydrated. After that, I simply waited it out and did what I could to help him recover.

I tried feeding him anything and everything, but he had no interest whatsoever in food. Bullet lost 15 pounds during those two weeks, dropping from 85 pounds to 70. I have no doubt that the discovery of Bully's Frozen Food Diet saved his life (see "Feeding Frozen," page 68).

I discovered one other method to get Bullet to eat—I don't have a clue how I came across it. I place the food bowl within Bullet's reach and I insert a finger into his ear (sometimes one in each ear) and rub gently, back and forth. Where? Somewhere within the nooks and crannies. I discovered a particular spot that seems to prompt a reflexive eating response! I make no guarantees, but perhaps it will work with your dog, too.

After Bullet's first dramatic weight loss, I made a decision to KEEP HIM FAT, and this remained a mantra throughout. I tried to maintain him at about five pounds over what I considered to be his perfect weight. My thinking was that I would not panic about a one- or two-day fast if he had a few extra pounds on him.

Vomiting was not a problem for Bullet. He vomited once after about one-third of the chemotherapy sessions and two or three times after a few of the chemotherapy treatments. The vomitus usually consisted of a large volume of clear fluid, which I cleaned up as best I could.

Bullet lost all of his whiskers at months 3 of his chemotherapy protocol, but the rest of his coat remained intact until month 17. At that time, with only one month of chemotherapy left, his entire undercoat fell out suddenly, in handfuls. For the first time in his life, Bullet was showing pink skin on his belly.

I added supplements that are said to promote hair growth to his regimen and the undercoat grew back nicely. Then, his guardhair coat dropped out. His head and neck retained the double coat typical of a Northern breed dog, but the rest of his body was furred only with a soft, downy undercoat. The next time we went to Dr. Porzio's office for a chemotherapy treatment, the doctor saw Bullet and exclaimed, "The Bullet looks like a giant chinchilla!"

Now, two years later, Bullet still has no guardhair coat except around his neck. I do miss watching my fingers disappear into Bullet's deep, luxurious fur but, all in all, I know that this is a very small price to pay.

References

1 Data collected from:
a) *Small Animal Clinical Oncology*, editors Stephen J. Withrow, DVM, diplomate ACVIM (oncology) and E. Gregory MacEwen, VMD, diplomate ACVIM (oncology and internal medicine). W.B. Saunders Company, 2001.

b) *Manual of Small Animal Internal Medicine*, by Richard W. Nelson, DVM and C. Guillermo Couto, DVM. Mosby, 1999.
c) *Veterinary Oncology Secrets*, editor Robert C. Rosenthal, DVM, PhD. Hanley & Belfus, Inc, 2001,

7

WHAT'S FOR DINNER?

Extensive research has been done toward understanding the relationship between nutrition and canine cancer. The consensus is that dietary intake is a significant factor in the survival of the cancer patient.

A great deal of what's known about the effect of diet on canine cancer is known due to the research of a veterinary oncologist at Colorado State University College of Veterinary Medicine and Biomedical Sciences. Gregory K. Ogilvie, DVM, diplomate ACVIM (Internal Medicine and Oncology), professor of Oncology and Internal Medicine, worked with his team at the veterinary college and a team from the Science & Technology Center at Hill's Pet Nutrition, Inc.® to develop Prescription Diet® Canine n/d®, currently the only commercial food formulated specifically for dogs with cancer.

The n/d diet was formulated according to Dr. Ogilvie's findings. Studies show that dogs with lymphoma in chemotherapy and dogs with nasal or oral cancer in radiation therapy who eat n/d have a significantly longer survival rate than those who eat other commercially produced dog foods. Very possibly, dogs with any type of cancer would benefit from n/d—other cancers have simply not been tested.

The current dietary guidelines for dogs with cancer are based on two of Dr. Ogilvie's findings. In broad strokes, these findings are: 1) Cancer cells readily metabolize carbohydrates and 2) Cancer cells are unable to metabolize fats. Because the goal is to feed the patient and not the cancer, we provide those nutrients that the patient is able to utilize and that cancer cells are unable to utilize (i.e., certain fatty acids) and withhold those that the cancer cells can utilize, thereby depriving the patient of those nutrients (i.e., carbohydrates). There's no question that the "cancer diet," high in Omega N-3 fatty acids and low in carbohydrates, improves a dog's prognosis and his chance of achieving remission or cure.

A high-fat diet contains oil additives high in Omega N-3 fatty acids. Flax seed oil, cod liver oil and fish oil are at the top of this list. Flax seed oil is highest in N-3 fatty acid content but contains Omega N-6 fatty acids, which are not beneficial when treating cancer. Note that when N-3 fatty acids are used nutritionally or in supplement form, antioxidants such as vitamin E should be given as well.[1]

A diet low in carbohydrates omits foods that contain sugar or starch such as fruits, some vegetables, most grains, potatoes and legumes. Dog biscuits are often high in carbohydrates, so if you feel that they are essential in maintaining your dog's quality of life, then choose a biscuit with a low carbohydrate content.

Cancer Cachexia (ka-KEX-ia) is a condition that often develops secondary to cancer. A cachexic dog experiences drastic and progressive weight loss regardless of the quality or quantity of food eaten. He becomes unable to metabolize nutrients and, eventually, reaches a state of severe malnutrition. Once cachexia has developed, it's often irreversible even if cancer treatment achieves a cure or a remission. There are varying opinions on this topic, but a low-carbohydrate, high-fat diet may decrease the likelihood of cancer cachexia developing.[2]

Cancer anorexia can also develop secondary to cancer. It's similar to cachexia in that the dog undergoes extreme weight loss, but in this case the weight loss is due to the dog's refusal to eat. Cancer anorexia is more easily reversible than cancer cachexia.

FEEDING NATURALLY

Dogs have been domesticated for over 14,000 years but the dog food industry has been around less than a century. Modern science stepped in to save caretakers time—to make feeding as simple, tidy and effortless as pouring pellets into a bowl. It's easier for us, but is it healthy for them?

Commercially produced dog foods may be comprised of poor quality ingredients cooked at extremely high temperatures, thus destroying much or all of the natural nutritional content. Nutrients listed on the product label are in the food only because they have been added back in after processing, in the form of synthetic additives. For those who wish to feed "dog food" to their dogs with cancer, Hill's n/d Prescription Canine Diet is the best choice.

There is an alternative. Today, more and more caretakers of dogs are choosing not to feed their pets canned or bagged food.

You can feed your dog "real" food—that is, whole foods as opposed to processed foods. You may be thinking of the warnings you've undoubtedly heard. *"Don't feed your pets table food—it may kill them!"* It may, or may not, depending of course on what you eat. I'm not suggesting that you feed your dog a diet of table scraps or serve him up a dish of whatever you and your family are having for breakfast, lunch and dinner.

A natural or "wild-type" diet does *not* mean feeding your dog the same diet that you eat. It means providing him with a diet that mimics what a dog (or a wolf, with an identical genetic makeup to the dog), eats in the wild.

The wild canine doesn't eat fruits and vegetables. The *truly* wild diet (as opposed to the wild-*type* diet) includes the stomach and intestines of the prey animal, which may contain fruits and vegetables that have been partially digested. In the wild-type diet, these foods are either pulverized (as in a food processor) or cooked so that they too are consumed in a partially broken-down state. A dog's digestive system may not, in any case, have the ability to extract nutrients from these foods unless they are finely minced or cooked.

Wolf biologist L. David Mech states that the stomach of the prey is rarely eaten by the predator wolf. In spite of this finding, most wild-type canine diets do include pulverized or steamed vegetables.[3]

As for meat in a truly wild diet, caribou, deer, mice and other animals are natural prey of the wolf. This includes muscle meat and organs, some cartilage and bone. As for food preparation, the canine hunter certainly doesn't build a fire and cook his kill—he eats it raw.

IS A RAW DIET SAFE?

The canine physiology has a digestive tract and digestive acids that enable the body to process raw meat. There is controversy regarding the canine's susceptibility to such bacterium as *salmonella* and *E. coli*. Some veterinarians believe that dogs are invulnerable to these "bugs" while others disagree. Still others claim that it's a moot point so long as the food is frozen before serving.

The raw meat in Bullet's diet was frozen before it was served. While I prepared Bullet's food, however, I sometimes gave him tidbits of fresh raw meat not yet frozen. In more than three years, he has never, to my knowledge, suffered any ill effects. Vegetables included in the wild-type diet are raw but are pulverized in a food processor.

Some dogs don't tolerate raw food and some caretakers don't feel comfortable serving it. Here again, the choice is yours. The practice of feeding raw meat to a dog is controversial. In general, as would be expected, traditional veterinarians are against it and holistic veterinarians are for it.

Bullet ate a raw diet throughout his cancer treatment with no ill effects. Bullet's raw diet can be easily revised to become a cooked diet. More than two years after Bullet's cancer diagnosis, he developed a serious heart condition. At that time, I switched him from a raw diet to a cooked version of the same diet.

I boiled, baked or broiled the meat and steamed the vegetables, added other ingredients and then froze the final product in freezer-bags or containers. The oils should not be heated—they can be added into the mixture and frozen, or they can be added to individual meals as they are served.

If you cook meat for your dog, broil or poach it in water and save the "gravy" produced in the process. Freeze the gravy in containers and then thaw as needed to pour over your dog's meals. After thawing, dispose of the solidified fats that will congeal at the top.

Bullet's cancer diet can be revised for a healthy dog simply by reducing the quantities of oil and adding carbohydrates (i.e., rice, potato, oatmeal, etc al). Before Bullet was diagnosed, I fed him a diet of meat, whole grains and vegetables, proportioned at one-third each. If you're the caretaker of a cancer-dog and a healthy dog, you might consider serving the same food to both, but adding cooked rice or any form of carbohydrate to one of the dishes at serving time.

HOW HARD CAN IT BE?

Preparing food for a dog is not as difficult or as time-consuming as you might think. Granted, it's more involved than pouring kibble into a bowl but it is, in fact, pretty simple. On the color pages of this book, you'll find a cookbook-type guide to my routine for preparing his highness' food. Follow it as closely or as loosely as you like.

An excellent diet for cancer-dogs that approximates a homemade version of n/d can be found online at [www.veterinarypartner.com]. At the main Web page, type into the search box: "Susan Wynn" and click "Search." If this fails, type the name into your favorite search engine.

If you change your dog's diet in any way, do so gradually. This applies regardless of whether you are switching from store-bought food to n/d, from kibble to home cooked or from home cooked to raw. Mix the new diet with the old, $^1/_4$ to $^3/_4$, for a week. Continue to increase the new and decrease the old by $^1/_4$ each week. At the end of the month, you can donate any remaining "pre-cancer" food to your local shelter.

WATER

A dog in cancer treatment may experience vomiting and/or diarrhea. Either, if extended or severe, can lead to dehydration. Monitor your dog's water intake and keep him well hydrated. Check for dehydration if you note any signs or if you note a decrease in your dog's water intake.

When Bullet was diagnosed with cancer, a very wise woman told me that although eating organic and drinking filtered water may not be necessary for everyone, these are essential components of beating cancer. I was skeptical at the time but her words have stayed with me and now, years later, ring true.

In most areas of the country, tap water is shown in periodic studies to be potable, or safe to drink, with acceptable levels of toxins. "Allowable" levels of impurities in water may be

---

LEADING A DOG TO... MEAT-JELLO?

Michael Penney's dog, Hobbes, was diagnosed with lymphoma in August of 2003. Michael discovered the following method of increasing Hobbes' fluid intake.

- ▸ Mix gelatin (or pectin) with water per directions
- ▸ Boil lean beef, chicken or turkey in a small amount of water to make a concentrated broth
- ▸ Add broth to gelatin and let cool
- ▸ Pour into ice cube trays and place trays in the freezer

Your dog may eat the solidly frozen cubes right out of freezer, or may prefer to let them thaw and drink the liquid. Meat-Jello helped to get Hobbes to drink when he was reluctant to, and provided a bit of nutrition as well.

Printed by permission of Michael E. Penney, Holliston, MA.

tolerated by a dog or person with a healthy immune system, but for a cancer patient, filtered water is a must.

The simplest method of providing your dog with filtered water is to purchase a countertop filter and place it right over your dog's water bowl. Just open the spigot and fill the bowl. A more sophisticated (and expensive) method involves the installation of a whole-house water filter. A state of the art system will also include a reverse-osmosis filter that feeds into a separate spout at the kitchen sink. If you're considering installing a water-filtration system for your pup, plug into the "pro" column the fact that the whole family will benefit! For homeowners, a good filtration system is also a good investment and will be an attractive asset when you resell your house.

If your dog is dehydrated due to vomiting or diarrhea or if you feel he's not drinking enough fluid, try Michael Penney's solution to this problem (see "Leading a Dog to Meat-Jello," page 67).

FEEDING FROZEN

When a dog in cancer treatment stops eating, there is cause for concern. Reversing the "not eating" state of affairs is of the utmost importance even, if necessary, at the expense of breaking the cancer-diet rules. If your dog will not eat the foods that are recommended for cancer patients, then get him to eat foods that are not recommended.

During Bullet's first "flat out" episode, he stopped eating and showed no interest in food. He's always been a chunky guy and I didn't panic at first. I checked his temperature and found it to be 101.5 degrees, which is well within the normal range. I concluded that Bullet was nauseous—a chemotherapy side effect.I gave him anti-nausea supplements and remedies with no result.

After several days passed and Bullet had not eaten anything at all, I became alarmed. I was now determined to get him to eat. I held bits of meat to his lips, trying to push the limp things into his mouth with no success. I tried warming up the food, a method often suggested in this situation—no luck. After many attempts with different foods and different techniques, I finally found success.

Siberian Huskies are Northern dogs, sled dogs, happy eaters of frozen seal meat and the like. This mental image, combined with the realization that frozen food has little or no taste or smell and thus might be more palatable to a nauseous dog, prompted me to attempt the following.

I bought a bag of frozen smelt. I withdrew one smelt and held its pointed tail in the corner of Bullet's mouth, poised to give it a little push if his jaws opened. I applied only very gentle pressure...and waited. Eventually, his jaws opened slightly and I pushed a bit and again waited. Lo and behold, just when my fingers were about to become completely numb, a chewing reaction began!

For a few days, I periodically offered Bullet food in a bowl or out of my hand. When it became clear that he was not planning to eat on his own, I resorted to the "smelt in the corner of his mouth" method. After perhaps a week, probably when his gastrointestinal chemotherapy side effects diminished, the non-eating came to an end and Bullet returned to his normal eating habits.

If your dog isn't eating and you use the frozen fish method, get comfortable. It may take some time for his chewing reaction to kick in. If he tries to push the fish out of his mouth with his tongue, gently replace it in the corner of his mouth. He may become ticked off at your efforts—in this case, of course, stop trying. We hope that he will instead become tired of pushing it out and let it rest there. Eventually, you will see a reflexive chewing action begin. Frozen smelts saved the day many times during Bullet's cancer treatment.

After Bullet's appetite returned, he continued to eat frozen fish. I buy bags of Whiting and Pollack fillets (labeled "dressed" fillets) in the frozen fish section of the supermarket. These are not breaded and there is no sauce. They're just plain fish meat without head, skin and bones, ready to serve up raw-frozen, raw-thawed or cooked. Bullet still eats a frozen fish every day as a treat. I've also recommended frozen fish as treats to friends with dogs who do not have cancer and there have been very few rejections.

If your dog takes to eating frozen fish, you'll find this to be the simplest way imaginable to feed a dog. Toss a fillet straight from the freezer onto the porch or into the pen. No dishes to clean, nothing to mix, no muss, no fuss! So long as your dog eats the fillet while it's still frozen, there will be no fish residue or odor on the floor. Not so, however, for his breath. If you're in the habit of giving your dog kisses, I recommend that you wait a while after he eats a fish fillet, or else give his teeth a good brushing before your next smooch.

BULLET'S DIET

About once a month, I purchased ten to twelve pounds of organic beef and then spent a couple of hours preparing it. I bought any cut that the butcher was willing to discount, generally in slabs but occasionally ground. Bacterium contaminate beef much more quickly after it's been ground. Therefore, it's important to purchase, prepare and freeze ground beef as soon as possible after it's been ground.

My recipe was never the same from one month to the next. Always included, however, were: Beef, chicken or turkey; flax seed, salmon and cod liver oils; broccoli, tomatoes and cabbage; eggs, tofu and garlic. Sometimes included were Brussels sprouts, broccoli sprouts, beef liver, beets, carrots and grapes.

After combining the meat with the vegetables and other ingredients, I scooped it into freezerbags, then placed these in the freezer. During the month, I thawed one bag in the refrigerator and when Bullet ate the last of that bag, I rotated another down from the freezer to the refrigerator.

There is no one combination of foods that you can feed your dog every time he eats and be certain that you are giving him the best foods to fight cancer. Hence, flexibility, variety and rotation are a good idea.

With the exception of a pound cake-and-pills combo, two dog biscuits daily and vegetables high in antioxidants, Bullet had virtually no carbohydrates for two years. No grains, potatoes, bread, cereal or foods containing high levels of sugar or starch.

BULLET'S DIET

Quantities are for approximately one week of fine dining for a 75-pound dog. Of the final frozen product, $3/4$ is meat and $1/4$ is vegetables. At feeding time, I sometimes added Hill's n/d as about $1/4$ of the total meal so that Bullet would be familiar with the taste.

Use organic foods whenever possible and always give a cancer-dog filtered water. A countertop filter can be positioned with its spigot above the water bowl.

INGREDIENTS

Beef, chicken or turkey..3 pounds
Tomatoes 2
Cabbage...$1/4$ head
Broccoli floret, some stem..2
Eggs (yolks raw, whites cooked)...3
Tofu ....$1/4$ lb
Salmon oil; Cod liver oil; Flax Seed oil: ....6 Tbs
Hulled or cracked Flax Seeds ....1 Tbs
Garlic ....3 - 4 cloves

TREATS

Frozen Whiting or Pollack fillet............................1 - 2/day
    (Frozen smelts can be substituted for small dogs)
Frozen-then-thawed RAW chicken wing 1/day
Plain organic yogurt...............................1 small bowl/day
Chopped up broccoli or string beans............on demand
"Cheese bone" 1/day
    (Hollow beef bone, press cheese into it)
Raw frozen beef bone 1/day

BULLET'S DIET

A Sampling of Ingredients

Tomatoes Cabbage Kale

Garlic   Oils

Tofu   Broccoli   Carrots   Eggs   Meat

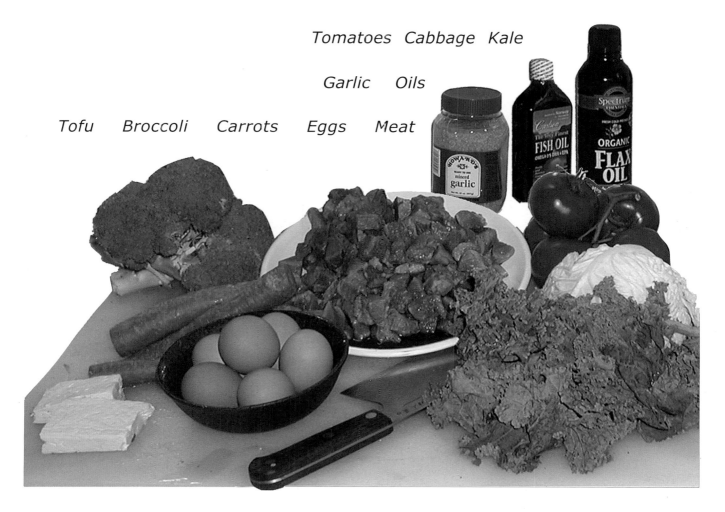

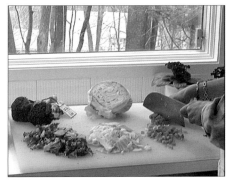

1. "Dry" Vegetables

Use broccoli and a cabbage-family vegetable. Kale, celery, carrots and other vegetables can be used as well.

Steam or food-process vegetables. Set aside.

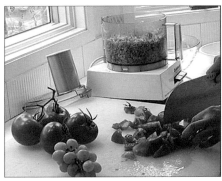

2. "Wet" Vegetables

Always use tomatoes. Grapes are controversial—include sparingly.

Steam or food-process vegetables. Add to vegetable bowl.

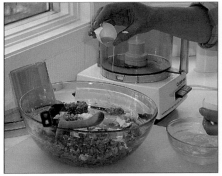

3. Egg Yolks

Add yolks into the vegetable bowl. Drop whites and crumbled shells into another bowl to be cooked.

Cook egg whites and crumbled egg shells—they may deplete biotin.

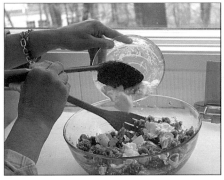

4. Egg Whites and Shells

Cook the whites and crumbled shells until the egg-white is solid enough to cut with a fork.

Add to vegetable bowl.

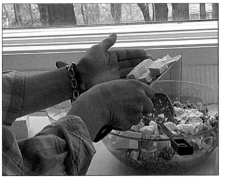

5. Tofu

Tofu is a very good source of protein. It may be added into the combination at any point of the process.

After adding all ingredients except meat and oils, hand mix as though tossing a salad.

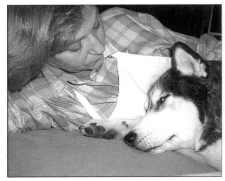

6. Take a Break!

If your dog works as hard as Bullet does, he's likely exhausted by now.

You can divide your work into two parts by stopping at this point—just cover and refrigerate the bowl overnight.

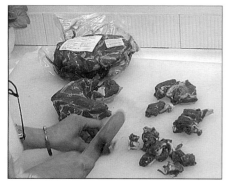

7. Prepare Meat

Cube the meat into bite-sized pieces. Use beef, chicken, turkey or fish. Meat may be cooked or raw.

Put cubed meat into a bowl and retrieve the vegetable bowl from the refrigerator.

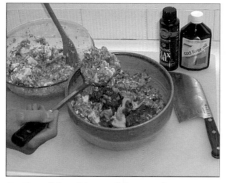

8. Combine Vegetables and Meat

Add processed or cooked vegetables to the meat so that about ¼ of the contents is vegetable and ¾ is meat.

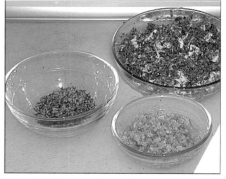

9. Add Flax Seeds and Garlic

Add flax seeds (be sure they're hulled or milled) and garlic.

Add about 1 tsp flax seeds and about a clove of garlic per pound of meat.

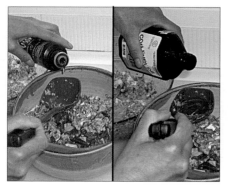

10. Add Oils

Use about 2 Tbs of oil per pound of meat.

I don't actually measure—I add oils after combining the meat with the vegetables and I watch to see how much oil the meat absorbs.

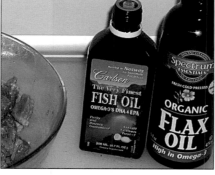

11. Vary Types of Oils

Flax seed oil, fish oil, salmon oil, cod liver oil and olive oil are all high in Omega N-3 fatty acids. I recommend a rotation.

I used flax seed oil most consistently throughout Bullet's cancer treatment.

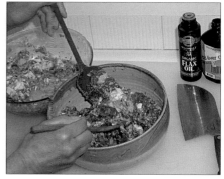

12. Hard Mix (toss) all

This is another good stopping point. If necessary, you can cover and refrigerate the bowls overnight.

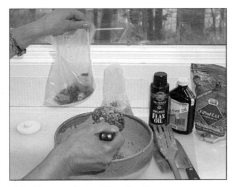

13. Scoop into Plastic Bags

Each storage bag should contain no more than three days worth of food.

Whenever you finish a bag, move another from the freezer into the refrigerator.

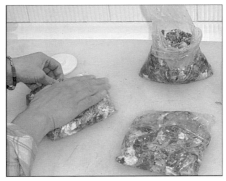

14. Flatten Bags

Frozen food should not be exposed to air. After filling a bag, squeeze the air out of it and pat it down flat.

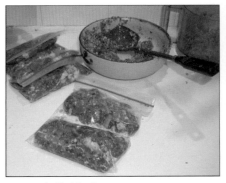

15. Subdivide bags

Depending on the size of your dog and of the meals he eats, you might want to subdivide bag contents.

When subdividing, use bags with air-tight closures, not fold-over sandwich bags.

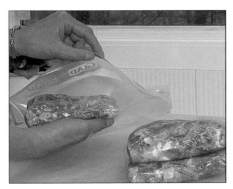

16. Double-Bag It

Keep bags free of air and the freezer free of drippings—pack small bags into a large one with air-tight closure.

If you're double-bagging, sandwich bags work fine for the inner package.

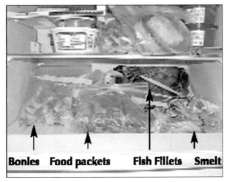

Bones   Food packets   Fish Fillets   Smelt

17. Freeze It

The bottom shelf of my freezer belongs to Bullet. Some dogs come running when they hear the sound of a can opener. Not my Bullet—he comes running to the sound of the freezer door opening.

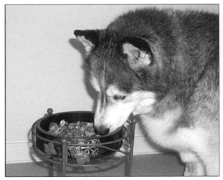

18. Thaw and serve!

At serving time, add n/d, yogurt, cottage cheese and/or supplements and medications.

Add filtered or bottled water to food if your dog isn't drinking enough water.

BULLET'S PHOTO GALLERY

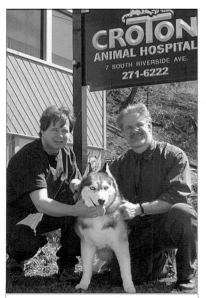

Vet tech Ed Mowan, Bullet and Dr. Bruce Hoskins.
He's in very good hands.

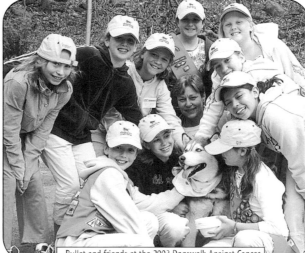

Bullet and friends at the 2003 Dogswalk Against Cancer

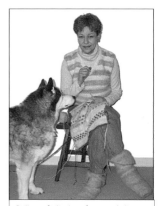

Bully-craft display of vest and slippers
(worn) and sweater (a work in progress).

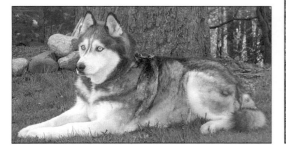

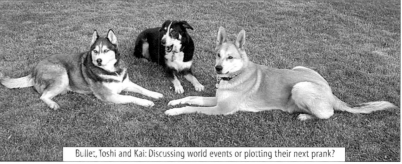

Bullet, Toshi and Kai: Discussing world events or plotting their next prank?

HOBBES

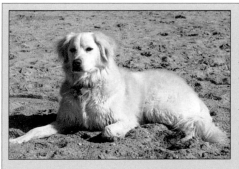

Mid-July 2003, Hobbes had a fluid-filled cyst removed from between his shoulder blades. The cyst, which turned out to be benign, could have resulted from an engorged tick that was removed about a week prior.

Hobbes crashed badly around August 4, 2003 and was rushed to the Foster Small Animal Clinic at Tufts. His diagnosis was 4b T cell lymphoma.

Hobbes' calm and reflective manner has been an 8-year lesson to me. Hobbes went to rest on Thursday April 22, 2004.

Michael Penney ~ Holliston, MA

MAX

Max is 6 years old and was diagnosed with Lymphoma in October 2002. He has undergone the Madison/Wisconsin chemotherapy protocol twice and has done very well. He loves to run in the country and play in the snow.

Mike & Kari Haislet,
~
Waterloo, Iowa

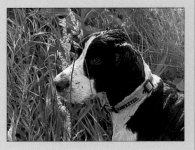

SUZI

Suzi is our beautiful 13-year young Golden Retriever, diagnosed on January 22, 2004 with extranodal lymphoma. She had enlarged lymph nodes in her neck and cancer ulcers on her lips and tongue. Our initial decision was to not go the chemo route. She was 13, after all...how much more time could we have with her in any case? But Suzi's lymph nodes were growing and her veterinarian put her on prednisone, which shrunk the nodes immediately! We saw the holistic doctors at Smith Ridge Veterinary Center. There, Suzi was treated with chemo and supplements and cryosurgery was performed on her lips and tongue.

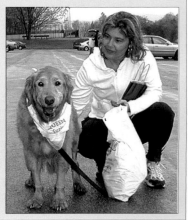

Suzi is now on the "cancer diet"—high fat, high protein, low carbs. She takes prednisone, lymph, BHI lymph, Mycel A, Artemisimim, Cell Advance, Rehmamia-6, Poly MVA and levothyroxine for her thyroid. This all seems to work—she was in remission by April 1, 2004. We stopped chemo then, but began again on May 27, 2004 when we noticed a suspicious growth on her lip.

One important thing I've learned over the past several months is that if your dog has cancer, no matter what treatment decisions you make, it will be the right choice for you and your dog. There is never a right or wrong decision!

Suzi is like our third child. She is gentle and loving and the joy of our lives. If you met her you'd know immediately why she is so special to us. She melts your heart!

Laurie & Kevin Hannon ~ Middletown, NY

MONA

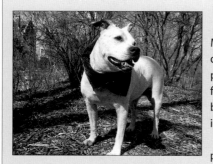

Mona's an 11-year-old pit mix. She was diagnosed in November 2003 with lymphosarcoma. She also tested positive for the disease in her liver and spleen, but not in her bones. She was becoming listless and obviously ill.

We started Mona on a rigorous supplement regimen under the instruction of a vet trained in eastern medicine and modified her diet to reduce carbs and increase protein. We also began chemotherapy with a veterinary oncologist. Mona was in remission within a week of the first treatment and had six chemo treatments over six weeks. We had to stop chemo treatments due to finances.

Mona is still taking herbal supplements and is still under the care of her general veterinarian for monitoring. She's holding remission after six months and is very healthy and happy. Although we are very grateful for her current condition, it did not come without a price—emotionally and financially. Online support groups, veterinary advice, and internet resources are invaluable. No, it's not an easy path, but yes, it's definitely worth it. Just look at her happy face!

Dawn Petrlik ~ Brooklyn, NY

DROOPY

On July 5, 2003, I was rubbing Droopy's head and floppy ears when I discovered enlarged lymph nodes on his neck. Within 48 hours, the nodes doubled in size. Droopy was diagnosed with stage III to IV lymphoma. He started chemo and natural therapies and went into remission after 5 weeks. A week later, he relapsed.

About two months later, Droopy died. When he took his last breath, I knew that he was not going to take another and I felt such a peaceful feeling from him as he left me to cross the rainbow bridge.

Droopy fought a brave and valiant battle like a trooper against lymphoma for 4 months and became a furangel on November 3, 2003.

Patricia Brown ~ Columbia, SC

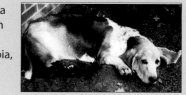

KIMMY

Kimmy's a 6^1/$_2$-year-old female beagle. She was diagnosed with lymphoma on March 7, 2003, at the age of 5^1/$_2$. Kimmy was treated with the 25-week Madison/Wisconsin chemotherapy protocol. She achieved remission quickly with no side effects and completed the protocol in mid-August 2003. In mid-November 2003, Kimmy came out of remission and is currently repeating the same protocol, except that Mitoxantrone is being substituted for Doxorubicin.

Kimmy acheived a second remission with 24 hours of her first treatment and has been doing very well. She will remain on maintenance chemotherapy this time for indefinite period.

Maureen

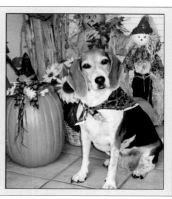

DIAMOND DREAMER

I was playfully giving Diamond Dreamer a belly massage when I first felt them: enormous lumpy bumps. My first thought was breast cancer, although she had been spayed before turning six months old. I rushed her to the vet on January 26, 2004, where she had blood work and biopsies. The verdict left me spinning in disbelief—Diamond had lymphosarcoma. How could this healthy, happy Labrador mix who was never ever sick have cancer? I had sworn against chemo after seeing it prolong my mother's ovarian cancer, but could I stand to lose my precious pooch in 30 days?

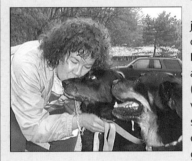

After tons of research and joining a wonderful pet cancer support group on the Internet, I decided to go with a combination of chemo (administered by a holistic veterinarian) and nutritional supplements along with a diet of raw meats and veggies.

If your dog has been diagnosed with cancer, draw upon your inner core of strength to research, as knowledge is indeed power. Diamond is more than halfway through her chemo protocol. Although the nodes balloon and then slowly deflate, I'm grateful that she has had no side effects except for one scary breathing episode.

No one can believe that Diamond is a cancer patient. She hikes and swims, eats with passion and has a gorgeous glossy coat. She's my wizard of mirth, and with her tireless tick-tock tail and winking amber eyes, she has taught me how to enjoy today's sunshine. Diamond is my Velcro dog, and I'm blessed each day she shares her happy spirit with me, her canine brother Splash Kisser, and our rabbit quintet.

Nancy Furstinger ~ Elizaville, New York

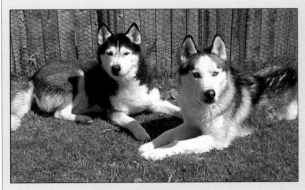

NATASHA

We are always very proud of our old girl Natasha (above left at 11 years old), who valiantly struggled with and successfully fought off the cancer for three years, after an initial prognosis of just 30 to 60 days!

Below, Natasha's 13th birthday party on April 21, 2001. This was her last birthday with us. Shilo and Jesse, the other pet cancer survivors whose stories are outlined on the Web site, are both still alive and cancer free today.

Please visit our Web site with Natasha's Cancer Fight Newsletter. Use any search engine and enter the words Natasha, Cancer and Fight.

Ron Conley
&
Family

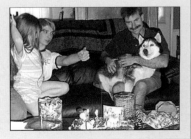

I honestly didn't think Bullet would live long enough to suffer any consequences because of a carbohydrate-deficient diet. Now that he has lived that long and longer, I do give him carbohydrates and he absolutely devours these foods, as though on some level he knows that he's been deprived of carbohydrates...which fits nicely with my herbalist's theory that Bullet self-medicates. Every night before bed, we each have a bowl of oatmeal and I often add brown rice to his meals.

VARIETY FOR LIFE

The most important benefit of feeding your dog a homemade diet rather than processed food is that he will be eating whole foods. An added benefit is that it's easier to provide nutritional variety. Serving the same old homemade meal twice a day every day negates this benefit.

Beef was the mainstay of Bullet's cancer diet, but periodically I substituted chicken or turkey—occasionally lamb or venison. I often cooked a bag of the same whiting fillets that he eats raw-frozen as a snack. Whenever salmon steaks or fillets were on sale, I prepared salmon as the "meat" portion of the meal to add variety to the diet. Tina Aiken, Bullet's holistic veterinarian, recommended that

I also include organ meat and ground bone in his diet. I recommend that cancer-dog caretakers do this, but I did not.

The core vegetables in Bullet's diet were those that are high in vitamin C and are thought to be important in an anticancer diet. They include tomatoes, broccoli and cabbage. Other vegetables high in Vitamin C can also be used. Include broccoli sprouts and any cabbage-family member (such as brussels sprouts and bok choy), kale, spinach, cauliflower, red peppers and garlic cloves. Use carrots and beets sparingly due to their high sugar content.

Pumpkin and squash are noted to be beneficial to cancer patients. Pumpkin in particular is also a good remedy for diarrhea. Grapes are included in many cancer diets for humans but are thought by some not to be good for routine canine consumption. By way of a compromise, I include grapes only occasionally in Bullet's diet.

DON'T FORGET THE TREATS

Most commercially produced dog treats are high in carbohydrates and are not on the "approved" list for our cancer-dogs' consumption. Still, our cancer pups should not be deprived of yummies! Quality of life includes being rewarded for good behavior and, in my book, survival is very good behavior. We simply need to be creative.

Try these cancer-healthy treats on your dog. If he isn't interested, be creative. Try anything he might like that doesn't contain sugar or starch.

TREATS

▸ Plain organic yogurt

▸ Cooked turkey or chicken meat, diced

▸ Raw, chopped vegetables. Try broccoli, string beans or carrots. Especially good for dogs who like crunchy treats. (Remember, not too many carrots because of the high sugar content.)

▸ "Cheese bones." These are easy to prepare. Just press a slice of cheese into the end of a hollowed out, marrowless beef bone. A cheese bone will keep a dog busy for a while, is refillable and dishwasher-safe.

FROZEN TREATS

I give Bullet the following treats raw-frozen. Any not otherwise noted can alternatively be served thawed-raw or cooked, but then they seem more like food items than treats and are not as much exercise for a dog's teeth and jaws.

▸ Hill's n/d (slide out of can, cube and freeze)

▸ Whiting or pollack fillets; smelts

▸ Chicken hearts

▸ Beef bones (soup bones)—MUST be raw!

▸ Whole chicken wings—MUST be raw!

▸ Turkey necks—MUST be raw!

References

1 *Natural Health Bible for Dogs & Cats,* by Shawn Messonnier, DVM. Prima Publishing, 2001, p.302.

2 *Veterinary Oncology Secrets,* editor Robert C. Rosenthal, DVM, PhD. Hanley & Belfus, Inc, 2001, p.107.

3 *The Wolf: The Ecology and Behavior of an Endangered Species,* by by L. David Mech. University of Minnesota Press, 1981.

8

WHAT ELSE CAN I DO?

You've decided on a medical plan, you're putting together a team of advisors and you have put a cancer diet into action. Now you're asking, *"What else can I do?"* It's time to add supplements to the home-care regimen.

Many supplements can be used in addition to or in some cases instead of traditional cancer treatment. Some natural remedies may protect your dog from the various ravages of chemotherapy, radiation or surgery.

Supplements claiming to fight cancer are, for the most part, untested. Your selection process will therefore be largely guesswork. Many veteran caretakers of cancer-dogs, holistic veterinarians and, of course, vendors believe that supplements play a crucial role in the fight against cancer. Many traditional veterinarians and some veteran cancer-dog caretakers say with equal certainty that few or none of the supplements that claim to fight cancer are effective.

Marlene Hauck, DVM, PhD, Assistant Professor, Oncology at North Carolina State University College of Veterinary Medicine, treats Buddy. This yellow Labrador Retriever appeared at the ACVIM's 21st annual Forum in 2003. At that time he was 9$\frac{1}{2}$ years old and had maintained a 6-year remission from lymphoma. In March 2004, Dr. Hauck was kind enough to answer a few of my questions about Buddy, as follows. (Dr. Hauck's responses are printed in italics.)

AN INTERVIEW WITH DR. HAUCK

What chemotherapy protocol and what other medical treatment was Buddy given?

Buddy received standard of care chemotherapy with a multi-agent, doxorubicin-based protocol. When he developed cardiotoxicity, the doxorubicin was changed to mitoxantrone. He received appropriate treatment for his cardiac disease as recommended by our cardiologists.

Did Buddy ever come out of remission?

Yes, he has come out of remission once so far.

Can you offer a hypothesis explaining Buddy's (and other survivors') very long survival of canine lymphoma?

Tumor heterogeneity. While we have prognostic factors for groups of animals, we cannot predict, at this time, how an individual patient will respond to treatment.

What sort of diet was Buddy fed?

Normal dog food. At one point, we considered putting him on a special diet for his heart, but I don't think we did so.

What supplements or alternative treatments did you or Buddy's owners provide?

Buddy did not receive any supplements or alternative treatments.

Is Buddy still alive?

Yes, Buddy is still alive.

Most veterinary oncologists that I've spoken to do not recommend "anticancer" supplements for their canine patients. According to Robert C. Rosenthal, DVM, PhD, diplomate ACVIM, diplomate ACVR, "Many owners are interested in complementary or alternative treatments, but none of these approaches have been shown to be of benefit for dogs with lymphoma. It is likely, but not a certainty, that most of these treatments will be innocuous." [1]

TO SUPPLEMENT OR NOT

Despite Buddy's longevity *without* the benefit of dietary and supplemental therapies, most cancer-dog caretakers I've interviewed want to cover all the bases just in case the supplements actually do give their dogs a better chance at survival. This is not a simple task. There's an endless list of pills, gel caps, capsules, powders, tinctures and teas that claim to fight or cure cancer. If you research in this area at all, you'll hear and read about many alternative treatments for cancer.

Give each due consideration but realize that no one has ever done *everything* that can be done for a cancer-dog. It's simply not possible to provide every medical treatment, every supplement and every alternative treatment. As the caretaker of a cancer-dog, you must draw the line where you need to and where it makes sense for you.

Choose alternative therapies carefully. Those that have not been scientifically, methodically tested in a controlled environment may or may not be effective. Some that seem to have merit may be worth adding if they're not too expensive and have been found not to have side effects or interfere with traditional treatment.

Remember to be fluid and flexible in your choices of supplements so that you can do each day what's best for your dog according to his current status and needs. From time to time, you might want to add in a new supplement and/or omit one that, in your mind, is less likely to be helping your dog fight cancer.

Few supplements, if any, have been sufficiently tested to inspire any certainty of efficacy. The lack of testing is in large part due to the astro-

DECISIONS YOU CAN MAKE

▸ **Consultants:** Choose your team members by referral or reputation and revise at will. The only goal is to have the strongest team possible.

▸ **Tests:** You have a great deal of say-so when it comes to testing. You can decline a test based on your dog's comfort level and the benefit to be gained by having the test. Gather information and consult with your team—the final decision is yours.

▸ **Leave or Wait:** If being left at the veterinarian's office is stressful for your dog, wait for the procedure and take him with you whenever possible. Remember, no one wants to be in a hospital longer than necessary—dogs included.

▸ **Shaving:** It's often necessary to shave some fur before surgery or chemotherapy, but generally not for a blood test. It's easier and quicker for the veterinarian but most will make the extra effort to draw blood without shaving if you so request.

Make every attempt to keep your dog intact and beautiful during treatment. It's easy to wind up with a patchwork dog, so keep the shaving to a minimum from the start.

You can specify which leg should be used for testing and treatment. If, for example, your dog is favoring a leg, you can request that a different leg be used for treatment.

▸ **Revisions:** If your dog isn't able to tolerate a treatment, ask your team members to suggest other options. There may well be another treatment that's equally effective and that your dog can better tolerate. If your dog is very ill, consider postponing the next treatment until he's stronger.

You're not at the mercy of any prescribed treatments, medications or schedules, but stick to the plan unless there's a reason to revise it.

nomical costs involved in performing the extensive testing required for FDA approval. Not many manufacturers of alternative health products can finance the testing and approval process.

Some testing has been conducted for many of the supplements, but on a smaller scale or without the controls necessary to qualify as FDA-level testing. The test population may be too small, dosages and frequencies not adequately controlled and/or the testing is not conducted as a double-blind test.

DON'T BLOW A FUSE!

In the summer of 2000, my kitchen counter was strewn with medication bottles. Each bottle was wrapped with a strip of masking tape with instructions written on it. BID, TID, with food, orally alone. TID 2 days before chemo to 2 days after, BID not before or after chemo...

I'd venture into the kitchen several times a day, scan the array of bottles, vials and powders and feel overwhelmed. As time went on, a routine developed. I periodically eliminated a supplement and a new one, keeping the list current and dynamic.

When you set out to develop a treatment plan for your dog with cancer, be realistic. Begin with a few supplements that you believe will be most effective. When you learn from a reliable source of a new supplement that's thought to fight cancer, add it to your list and omit any that have been found not to be effective.

There is a great deal of anecdotal information about the success of various cancer fighting formulations. Most are documented by physicians, veterinarians or people who have used the product. Many manufacturers will provide a list of testimonials from users of the product, either on their Web sites or in pamphlets.

The following section contains an overview of supplements commonly recommended for cancer-dogs. This is not by any means a comprehensive listing. Consult your veterinary oncologist, your holistic veterinarian and/or your health store advisor to establish which supplements to give your dog and in what amounts.

SLOW DOWN

There is an endless list of supplements that allegedly fight cancer. Some are known to offer benefits to the cancer patient and others are thought to help. You might be inclined to use all of them: Don't! You'll spend a great deal of money, become overwhelmed and traumatize your dog with constant pilling. Use restraint and discrimination and select 5 to 10 supplements to start out—choose the ones that you believe will be effective—then revise the list as needed.

Many dogs become reluctant to eat when they're ill, whether the illness if due to cancer, chemotherapy or some other, unrelated cause. If your dog is "off his foods" and you are working hard just to get some nutrition and essential medications into him, put aside any supplements that aren't working to heal his immediate condition until he is feeling better. Basic nutrition and the medications known to be effective are far more essential than the supplements that may or may not be effective.

Don't add supplements to your dog's regimen willy-nilly. Apart from the potential for cancer-fighting and immune system boosters to wipe out your savings account, apart from the certainty that you'll blow a fuse trying to keep it all straight (which to give when, how many times a day, with food or without, give only before and after chemotherapy or do not give within "x" days before or after chemotherapy) and apart from the possibility that the supplements you choose won't be effective, there is a more dangerous possibility.

Interactions can occur between supplements or between a supplement and a prescribed medication. Some supplements interfere with the intended activity of certain prescription drugs or chemotherapy agents. Regarding supplements that many cancer-dog caretakers give their dogs, Dr. Rosenthal says, "Reports of adverse reactions are beginning to surface, and clinicians should be aware that there are no good data on possible interactions of the alternative compounds often suggested in varied combinations, either with each other or traditional cytotoxic agents."[2]

Speak to your veterinarian and other owners of dogs with cancer. If your veterinarian isn't up to speed on supplements (and many are not), find a holistic veterinarian to consult in person or by telephone.

Dr. Cotter offers another good reason to choose supplements with caution: "I advise owners not to begin giving any new supplement to their dog while he is having chemotherapy treatments. The reason for this is that if the dog becomes ill, it's difficult to determine whether the illness is a reaction to the chemotherapy or to the supplement."

After deciding on a list of supplements that you want to include in your anticancer program, comparison-shop for the best prices at a health food store and on the Internet. Some supplement products also vary in quality from one manufacturer to another. Through companies such as Consumerlab.com, LLC, research the relative quality of supplements as produced by various manufacturers.[3]

VITAMINS AND MINERALS

Vitamins and minerals are fundamental to any dog's diet. When a dog is combating cancer, they are essential. Dr. Messonnier states: "Studies demonstrate that both people and pets with inadequate nutrition cannot metabolize chemotherapy drugs adequately.... This makes proper diet and nutritional supplementation an important part of cancer therapy."[4]

After deciding on a list of supplements to give your dog, ask your veterinarian or a veterinary nutritionist to look it over to find any conflicts or cumulative excesses. In 2001, at the recommendation of Dr. Ogilvie, I started giving Bullet Centrum Silver® daily. As a result, his entire supplement list had to be reviewed and revised.

SOME GENERAL GUIDELINES

▸ Vitamins A, C, D, E, K and beta-carotene are important supplements for cancer patients because of their antioxidant properties.
▸ Vitamin A in combination with beta-carotene may benefit patients undergoing chemotherapy, surgery or radiation for cancer.
▸ Vitamin E is thought protect against the ill effects of the chemotherapy agent doxorubicin while enhancing its effectiveness. Ask your veterinarian for the proper dosage as this vitamin.
▸ Zinc and Magnesium are thought to be helpful in the fight against cancer.
▸ If your dog is predominantly or fully a particular breed, ask your veterinarian if there are any deficiencies typical to that breed. For example, Huskies tend to be Zinc deficient.

Your dog gets some nutrients through his diet, whether it's a home-prepared diet or commercially produced dog food. How can you know which nutrients and in what quantities he needs in supplement form? A blood test called a Bio-Nutritional Analysis (BNA) can be preformed to determine the amount of each mineral and vitamin in a blood sample and to test organ functioning.

After reviewing the results of a BNA test, your veterinarian will advise you of any deficiencies found in your dog's test. You can then take steps to correct the imbalance. Veterinarians who recommend this test—in my experience only holistic veterinarians do—generally offer to provide a compounded supplement formulated especially for your dog according to the test results. If you're not prepared to take one of the following actions, there's little point in having a BNA test done.

CORRECTING IMBALANCES

▸ Your veterinarian may offer to have a powder made up for you that contains the vitamins and nutrients your dog needs, based on the results of the BNA test. You can purchase this as a powder or in encapsulated form.

▸ Adjust your dog's diet, adding foods rich in any deficient vitamin or mineral and omitting foods that exacerbate known weaknesses.

▸ Purchase all of the supplements needed at a health food store, from an herbalist or online.

OTHER SUPPLEMENTS

When you hear about a supplement that piques your interest, read up on it. Talk to veterinarians, other cancer-dog caretakers and people who have used the supplement. Don't forget to search the Net. After collecting your data, decide on a preliminary group of supplements that you believe in, and get started. Remember, you can revise this list at any time.

IMMUNE SYSTEM AND NK CELL BOOSTERS

Some chemotherapy protocols are highly immunosuppressive and there are varying theories about the wisdom of using antioxidants to boost the immune system when medical treatment is designed to suppress it. Be sure to discuss this with your veterinarian or veterinary oncologist before adding an immune-system booster to your dog's anticancer regimen.

Many supplements claim to boost NK cell (Natural Killer cell) activity and/or production. NK cells attack other cells that are unwanted invaders, such as cancer cells. When cancer is present and a dog's NK cells are fighting an ever-growing army of cancer cells, the supply of NK cells may be depleted. Clearly, any cancer patient would benefit from an increase in the number and activity of NK cells. The following represent NK cell boosters included in a home care regimen for a dog with cancer.

▸ **Astragalus:** This is available in several forms, including capsules, tinctures and ground root. It boosts the immune system and acts as an anti-inflammatory.

▸ **MGN-3** is made from rice bran and shiitake mushroom extracts. According to the manufacturer (Lane Labs), MGN-3 builds up B, T and NK (natural killer) cell components of the patient's immune system.

▸ **IP-6** is another NK cell booster. The information I've gathered indicates that MGN-3 is more effective in dogs.

ANTIOXIDANTS

There are quite a few vitamins, minerals and herbs that benefit cancer-dogs because of their antioxidant properties. Antioxidants turn free radicals (cells that are missing one electron) into healthy cells by adding the missing electron. Free radicals are precursors of cancer cells. In other words, free radicals are likely to become cancer cells if they are not converted into healthy cells through the addition of that missing electron.

You might want to consult your veterinary oncologist before giving antioxidants to your dog while he's in cancer treatment. Some studies indicate that supplementation with a very high level of antioxidants may actually be counterproductive—that it may actually help cancer cells to multiply.

Other studies show that antioxidants are not only safe, but are beneficial to dogs in chemotherapy. Some antioxidants are said to enhance the effects of certain chemotherapy drugs. Having a holistic veterinarian on your team is the best way to ensure that your dog is on the best antioxidant supplements in light of his medical treatment, other supplements and nutritional intake.

Many antioxidants have curative or protective effects on a particular organ or system. These are noted for each antioxidant in parentheses.

- **Vitamins** A, C, D, E, K, beta-carotene and selenium.
- **Black Currant:** Anti-inflammatory properties. (Skin)
- **Cordyceps:** Oxygenates the system. *Not to be used before surgery or with anticoagulants. (Lungs)
- **Coenzyme Q_{10}:** Can cause nausea at high doses. (Heart function; gum health)
- **Curcumin** (found in Turmeric): Anti-inflammatory properties. (Heart function)
- **Germanium Sisquioxide:** Oxygenates and dehydrogenates the body. *Give on alternate weeks—one week on; one week off, etc. (Many benefits)[5]
- **Glutathione:** An amino acid. Reduces damage to kidneys if used with chemotherapy agent cisplatin. Minimizes diarrhea when used with radiation therapy. (Immune system)
- **Green Tea extract:** Protects against effects of radiation exposure.
- **Hawthorne:** (Heart function)
- **Pycnogenol:** A mixture of bioflavonoids that may enhance the effects of vitamin C as an antioxidant. (Heart function)
- **Quercetin:** An antioxidant bioflavonoid. May enhance the effect of chemotherapy, radiation therapy and hyperthermia. (Allergies; asthma)

"CANCER FORMULAS"

A few of the many products that are said to fight cancer are included in this list. Most have only anecdotal evidence of success and provide no supporting scientific data.

- **Hoxsey's Cancer Formula:** May have cytotoxic and immunostimulating properties. Contains Berberine and other herbs.
- **Essiac Tea:** Burdock root, Sheep sorrel, Slippery Elm bark and Turkey rhubarb root. Acts as an antitumor antioxidant and immunostimulant.
- **Pau D'Arco** and **Cat's Claw:** Both anticancer herbs. Alternate weekly rather than giving both concurrently.
- **Poly-MVA™ (Polydox):** A palladium lipoic complex (LaPd) and DNA reductase containing nutrients that may be depleted during chemotherapy and radiation therapy. Polydox may encourage tumor reduction.[6]
- **Transfer Factors:** Created from naturally occurring polypeptides. Stimulates immune system function by enhancing the function of lymphocytes called T-Helper cells.[7]
- **Artemesia:** A Chinese herb that has killed cancer cells in a test tube.
- **Seacure:** Biologically hydrolyzed whitefish. A protein supplement with many benefits. May alleviate chemotherapy side effects.

ORGAN SUPPORT

Chemotherapy and radiation are toxic and damaging to body tissues. Toxins travel through the digestive tract, kidney and liver. You can strengthen these organs and systems as follows:

- **DIGESTIVE SYSTEM**

  L-Glutamine, an amino acid. "...Supports protein synthesis, improves gastrointestinal repair and regeneration, and augments both systemic and gastrointestinal immune response."[8] *Do not give your dog L-Glutamine if he has epilepsy or is taking antiseizure medication.*

  Acidophilus and **bifidus** are "good bacteria" found in the stomach but that be destroyed during chemotherapy. You can give this as a supplement in capsules or add organic yogurt with active cultures to your dog's daily diet. **Psyllium** husks powder cleanses the colon.

- **KIDNEYS**

  Digestive enzymes such as **Prozyme®** or **Wobenzyme®**; vitamin C.

- **LIVER**

  Milk Thistle detoxifies the liver. **SAMe** is protective. **L-Arginine** is an amino acid helpful in liver disease, heart disease and cancer and is included in n/d food. If you are not feeding your dog n/d, it's essential to provide this as a supplement.

SUPPLEMENTS WITH ANTIBIOTIC PROPERTIES

‣ **Bovine Colostrum,** a substance produced by a cow just prior to the production of mother's milk. Has powerful antibiotic properties. Available in powder or in encapsulated form.

‣ **Echinacea** defends primarily against upper respiratory infections.

‣ **Goldenseal** protects respiratory and digestive systems. This has antibiotic properties and stimulates the immune system.

ALTERNATIVE THERAPIES

Apart from the many supplements that can be given to a dog to help in his fight against cancer, there are treatment modalities that, although they will not cure cancer, may be beneficial.

ACUPUNCTURE

This ancient modality doesn't cure or treat cancer, but is used successfully during cancer treatment to alleviate side effects, support organs in need of fortification and generally balance body systems and energy flow.

Rodney Page, DVM, diplomate ACVIM (Internal Medicine; Oncology), is a professor at and the director of the Sprecher Institute for Comparative Cancer Research at the College of Veterinary Medicine at Cornell University. Dr. Page says, "Of the current alternative therapies, I believe acupuncture has the most solid evidence of benefit for the relief of neurogenic or orthopedic pain developing from cancer."

MASSAGE

If your dog enjoys massage (and who doesn't?), go for it! It will soothe him and will be a time for bonding. It may encourage circulation and healing and will allow you to discover new lumps or bumps early. When massaging a dog with cancer, some say that hand movements should travel away from the heart.

Myofascial release, Tellington Touch and other healing-touch techniques may also encourage healing, circulation and relaxation.

SYNCHRONIZED BREATHING

If your dog's breathing is labored, shallow or uneven, lay next to him (the spoon position works well). Synchronize your breathing to his and then very gradually shift your breathing to a deep, even pattern. You may hear your dog's breathing shift, trying to stay in time with yours. When you hear a deep, slow breath, a heavy sigh, a cleansing breath, your mission is accomplished.

BULLET'S SUPPLEMENTS

My experience with supplements for canine cancer occurred at our first appointment at Dr. Marty Goldstein's office. I left with a bag full of bottles, vials and boxes and with little understanding of what they were or how they worked.

As I gathered information, I revised Bullet's regimen many times. The cancer supplements that I gave Bullet and that I consider most important are named below. Regarding quantities, remember that Bullet weighed about 80 pounds.

▸ **Astragalus:** I discovered dried astragalus root in 2001. Slices of the root resemble tongue depressors and can be steeped in a soup, a stew or a cup of tea. One day, a slice of astragalus root fell to the floor on its way to my teacup and Bullet attacked it! He tossed it in the air, chased it down and devoured it entirely. I added this to my list of Bullet's treats.

Sometimes Bullet eats astragalus eagerly; at other times, he shows no interest in it. My herbalist believes that Bullet self-medicates—that he eats it only when his system requires it. I also sprinkle a three-finger pinch of shredded astragalus root on each meal that Bullet eats.

▸ **Colostrum:** As needed, if stools contain blood. This is a natural antibiotic.

▸ **L-Arginine:** 500 mg twice a day. If Bullet had been eating n/d, I would have given less.

▸ **L-Glutamine:** Beneficial to intestines and other body systems. I gave Bullet 1 tsp twice a day throughout his cancer treatment. I doubled the dose a few days before and after each treatment. When he had digestive or excretory problems, I doubled or tripled the dose.

▸ **MGN-3:** 500 to 1000 mg once a day. This replaced IP-6 about six months into Bullet's treatment.

▸ **Milk Thistle:** ¼ tsp twice a day starting several days after treatment, for about three days. My herbalist sent packets of wild-crafted dried milk thistle seeds, which I ground in my coffee grinder and added to Bullet's pound cake-and-pill mix.

▸ **Poly MVA:** I gave Bullet a much lower dose of this supplement than is recommended by the manufacturer: 2 ml twice a day. I also put a few drops on any suspicious lumps and bumps that I found.

▸ **Antioxidants:** Cordyceps, CoQ_{10}, Germanium, Quercetin and Pycnogenol (in rotation). Also Vitamins C and E.

▸ **Other:** Multivitamin and B complex.

ASSESSING SUCCESS

Be careful not to assess the quality of care that you provide for your dog according to the number of months or years that he survives. Some people can't resist turning the longevity and survival rates of dogs with cancer into a competition.

Success stories about other dogs may be told with good intentions but can make one whose dog survived only a short time feel as though they failed to perform or to provide adequate care.

Stories about the passing of a cancer-dog or failure of treatment are not only sad in their own right but also fill us with trepidation: *More likely than not, my dog will be going down that road too sometime soon.*

It's not a race, folks. We don't yet know how to beat cancer. For those whose dogs survive longer than expected, there's no certainty of what it was that enabled them to survive. Nor do we know why some canine cancer patients don't respond to treatment. So just do your best and leave your competitive spirit at the gym!

References

1   *Veterinary Oncology Secrets*, editor Robert C. Rosenthal, DVM, PhD. Hanley & Belfus, Inc, 2001, p. 184.
2   ibid, p. 184.
3   www.consumerlab.com
    Phone: (914) 722-9149
4   *Natural Health Bible for Dogs & Cats*, by Shawn Messonnier, DVM. Prima Publishing, 2001, p.45.
5   *Germanium: Its Miracle Healing Effects and Health Implications*, by Yang Hwan Oh. Dorrance Publishing Company, 2003.
6   AMARC Enterprises
    Phone: (866) 765-9682
    Website: [www.polymva.com]
7   [www.vet4life.com]
8   *Veterinary Oncology Secrets*, p. 107.

9

WHOLE HEALTH

Imagine that your dog survives cancer for six months or a year and your veterinarian finds that his teeth are in need of extensive dentistry. Most dental work requires anesthesia and involves a chance of infection—two things that any dog would be better off without, but particularly a dog who is fighting cancer. It's important to remember that health and medical issues are no less likely to occur to your dog than they are to a dog without cancer.

Keep your dog in tip-top condition while he's fighting cancer. Any neglected health issue can lead to unnecessary complications. Vitamin and mineral deficiencies, for example, can undermine any dog's strength. For a dog with cancer, the repercussions can be more severe and more difficult to resolve.

The emotional upheaval of finding that your dog has cancer, combined with the logistical complexities of providing cancer treatment, can be overwhelming. Depending on the complexity of your dog's cancer treatment and home-care plan, you may have your hands full. Incidentals such as bathing, grooming and brushing his teeth may fall by the wayside.

The home-care tasks directly related to cancer will become routine before long and will require less of your time. Once this occurs, it's very important to reinstate a sound whole health home-care program. Elderly folk quip, "If I knew

I was going to live so long, I would have taken better care of myself!" Let's be optimistic and believe that your dog will live long enough, despite cancer, to benefit from your continued attention to his whole health.

During the course of cancer treatment, your dog may be immunosuppressed and therefore less able to ward off illness. When any secondary or unrelated health problem arises, find out what the treatment options are. Any veterinarians or specialists that you see should be aware of your dog's cancer status—the standard treatment for a particular illness may not be appropriate for a dog who also has cancer.

If a secondary illness occurs, contact all of your cancer team members to ask their recommendation. Consider all treatment options offered by all factions—allopathic, autopathic, holistic, herbal, homeopathic, naturopathic...and then decide on a course of action.

WEAK SPOTS WITH CANCER

Be vigilant for certain health problems in your cancer-dog. A weekly home-care checkup is the best way to sidestep secondary illnesses and keep your dog healthy and strong during treatment.

TUMORS

Check your dog's body for tumors regularly. This is very easy to do while you're giving him a massage. If you find any new lumps or bumps, inform your veterinarian.

Just two months after Bullet was diagnosed with lymphoma, Dr. Porzio examined a very small, pink pimple-like growth near Bullet's ear. He said it had the appearance of a benign tumor, and that we should watch it for any increase in size or change in appearance.

The tumor remained unchanged for a year but then suddenly grew to twice its original size. Dr. Hoskins removed it surgically as planned, using a short-acting anesthesia. One year later, another, similar tumor developed at the base of Bullet's ear and was removed. The laboratory report on the excised tissue stated that these were both benign tumors.

TEETH

When a dog is in cancer treatment, dental hygiene is especially important. Chemotherapy can be destructive to teeth and gums and it's always better not to subject a dog with cancer to dental surgery.

Chewing on bones is good for a dog's teeth. Even so, time will take its toll on tooth enamel and gums just as it does on humans even though we brush twice a day. To avoid traumatic (not to mention expensive) dental cleanings and dental treatments, brush those pearly whites!

Brush your dog's teeth every other day. Be sure to use a toothpaste made for dogs or for human infants—one without any fluoride. A small amount of fluoride is good for our teeth, but it's actually a poison. People are capable of spitting out rather than swallowing, but dogs (and babies) are not. Toothbrushes for dogs are sold at pet-supply stores; a child's toothbrush will work as well. There are toothpastes available for dogs and you can also use toothpastes that are intended for a baby's teeth.

Brushing the fronts of your dog's teeth is sufficient. I know very few dogs good natured enough to allow the inside surfaces of their teeth to be brushed.

If your dog isn't cooperative when you attempt to brush his teeth, introduce him slowly. Settle him down, show him the brush, lift his lip and make one quick stroke across his teeth. Give him a treat immediately. Do this one or more times a day, gradually upping the number of strokes each time. Most dogs become agreeable to the procedure quickly, especially if you find a flavored toothpaste that they like.

Eating frozen food may also be beneficial to a dog's tooth and gum health. I've seen no research on this subject.

ELBOWS

Include a check for elbow sores in your routine whole-health checkup—the sores that dogs tend to develop from sleeping on hard surfaces. If you find such a sore, toss area rugs or mats over any hard surfaces on which your dog snoozes. If you suspect that the sores are infected (foul smelling, full of pus or hot to the touch), inform your veterinarian right away.

I doused Bullet's elbow sores with hydrogen peroxide and applied an antibiotic ointment. I then either applied a wrap to prevent him from licking the medicine off, or I applied the medicine immediately before a walk or a feeding.

NAILS, PADS AND FEET

During chemotherapy, a dog's nails may become brittle and crack easily. Because nails are constantly growing, they are subject to the ill effects of chemotherapy.

In August 2001, Bullet and I were out hiking and I noticed that he was leaving bloody paw prints on the ground. I examined his feet to find that a nail had cracked off very close to its sheath.

SUPPORT YOUR DOG IN EVERY WAY THAT YOU CAN

by Dr. Allen M. Schoen

A comprehensive approach to fighting canine cancer should include a holistic, integrative component. The benefit of this approach is that it considers the dog's whole being, not just a particular tumor or cancer condition. Tend to the health of your dog's mind, body and spirit throughout and you will make him as strong as possible in order to help him in his fight against cancer.

Fascinating research shows that your attitude and intention may well impact on your dog's health. I suggest to my clients whose kindred spirits have cancer that they try not to express sadness and shed tears in the presence of their dog. Remain cheerful and loving in your dog's presence. This will be helpful to both of you.

Explore your attitudes towards your dog's condition. You may experience sadness, anxiety and fear of loss as you deal with the treatment of your dog's cancer. You should have a good support system to help you process the emotional challenges of helping your dog.

When fighting cancer, there is no one perfect approach for all dogs.

Include, as an integral part of your team, a veterinarian who is knowledgeable about the most recent advances in nutritional and botanical supplements. This person should be open to a comprehensive, integrative approach to cancer treatment.

Appropriate, balanced, natural nutrition is the foundation for any animal. Nutritional supplements and botanical medical supplements may be beneficial as a complementary approach above and beyond a dog's basic nutritional needs.

Some supplements help by counteracting potential side effects of chemotherapy and radiation therapy; others may be contra-indicated when using chemotherapy or radiation. Some supplements have been found to be therapeutically supportive in treating dogs with cancer and others actually are anticarcinogenic.

New supplements are constantly emerging as research documents the efficacy of various ones. This book describes excellent supplement regimens that will provide additional support to a dog with cancer.

As caretaker, your goal is to help your dog with cancer be as healthy and as happy as possible. You can incorporate all of the beneficial approaches to fighting cancer that are introduced in this book. In some cases, you can also help by relieving the pain that is associated with some cancers.

The key is to have your veterinary team working together to provide the best integrative approach possible to help your dog heal and remain healthy and happy.

In the Chinese language, the character for crisis is the same as the character for opportunity. This crisis can also be an opportunity to learn and your kindred spirit can be an excellent teacher.

Our canine friends can be wonderful teachers of love and compassion. We can use these opportunities to become blessings of love to all other beings and to be of great benefit to all creatures great and small.

Allen M. Schoen, MS, DVM, is author of Kindred Spirits, How the Remarkable Bond between Humans and Animals Can Change The Way We Live.

Once home, I pushed the open end of the nail into a bar of soap to stop the bleeding. Three more nails cracked off during the following month but then the cracking ended. I increased the egg and tofu content of Bullet's diet to provide more protein, rubbed Musher's Secret® into his nails and pads once a day and kept his nails clipped short.

Since Bullet wasn't hiking and running as he did in his pre-cancer days, the fur between his toes grew long enough to cover the pads. This made for a slippery walking surface, evidenced by Bullet's difficulty in ascending the ramp to the car. Keeping the fur between his toes clipped short gives him better traction.

HAIRCOAT

Because cancer cells divide more frequently than do healthy cells, chemotherapy agents are designed to attack cells that are in the process of dividing. As planned, the agents attack cancer cells, but healthy cells that happen to be in the process of cell division are also targeted.

The reason people in chemotherapy often lose hair is that the protein-based cells such as hair and nails undergo cell division at a higher rate than other cells. Dogs in chemotherapy, however, do not typically lose their "hair" because while the hair-growth pattern in humans is constant, it is seasonal in dogs. Don't forget to keep your dog's coat in good condition by bathing and grooming regularly.

It's common for dogs in chemotherapy to lose their whiskers. Bullet lost all of his whiskers three months after beginning treatment and a few months after his last chemotherapy treatment, new whiskers appeared. These are somewhat scraggly, but Bullet doesn't seem to mind.

Eighteen months after beginning treatment, Bullet lost his guardhair coat all at once. My herbalist recommended a supplement called Silica and provided me with dried, ground nettles to sprinkle on his food. The fallout ended but Bullet's guardhair coat has never returned. He still has a beautiful coat but it's shorter, fluffier and softer than the typical Husky coat.

STRESS AND PILLING

Common sense tells us that stress is not good for a dog with cancer. Watch your dog for signs of stress. Every dog has a different set of stressors just as each of us has a unique set of stressors—different, unique ways of manifesting stress and individual tolerance levels for stress.

When a dog is ill, pilling can become stressful, especially when there are many pills that are to be given over a long period of time. Putting a handful of medications and supplements down Bullet's throat three times daily would have been stressful for both of us.

▸ **Food-Plus-Meds:** If your dog is eating reliably, simply mix the pills that are not marked "on an empty stomach" with his food. However, there may be times when your dog isn't eating reliably, possibly due to treatment side effects. During these times, you may find yourself disposing of a great deal of uneaten food, along with medications. There are several ways to remedy this frustrating and expensive situation. Your dog's preferences may determine which method you choose.

▸ **PB&P:** Spread peanut butter or soy butter onto a bit of bread, press the pills into it, then fold it over to make a "peanut-butter-and-pills sandwich." If your dog is skilled at eating the bread and the spread and spitting out the pills one by one, try another method.

▸ **Pound Cake Plus:** Mix the pills and powders in a bowl with a bit of crumbled pound cake. This was our method of choice. Even when Bullet wasn't eating reliably, I could almost always persuade him to eat the pound cake-plus-meds combo.

An added advantage of using the "pound cake plus" method is that if your dog doesn't eat the offering, it's very easy to pick the pills out and try again later. Once pills have been mixed into a food bowl, they are difficult or impossible to retrieve.

▸ **Mix Powder with Water:** Use a needle-less syringe to mix the powder with filtered water. With a finger on the open end, shake to mix. Place the open end inside your dog's lips and slowly empty the contents into his mouth. Many supplements are available in powder form rather than encapsulated. If this method works with your dog, buy the powder form when possible.

▸ **Manual Pilling:** There were times when I could not get Bullet to eat the pills no matter what. In these cases, I "pilled him" manually.

MANUAL PILLING

▸ Stand next to your dog.

▸ With the hand nearest him, reach over his neck and under his chin. Insert your thumb and middle finger between his teeth, on either side of his lower jaw, to the rear of his "fangs."

▸ Gently but firmly pull down to open his jaw and, with your other hand, place the medications on his tongue, as far back as you can.

▸ Let his mouth close but hold his head up a bit and stroke his neck until he swallows.

WARDROBE

Since your dog's lymphatic system may play a role in his disease, it makes sense to avoid any irritation of his lymph nodes. Most dog collars press close to or directly over the submandibular nodes. Walking harnesses are preferable to collars even for a healthy dog, in order to avoid the development of tracheal collapse.

Many harnesses cut in closely behind the front legs, applying pressure to the prescapular nodes. I've found two lymph node-friendly harnesses: The Hug-a-Dog harness from D3Pet Productions (an open mesh, very cool on hot summer days) and the 3-in-1 Vest Harness from RC Pet Products (see "Resources" for contact information).

VACCINES AND CANCER

In *Natural Health for Dogs & Cats,* Dr. Pitcairn warns that, "Giving a vaccine to an animal with cancer is like pouring gasoline on a fire."[1] Dr. Dodds reports that the dog's immune system may compromised by vaccination for up to 45 days and, in the case of rabies vaccine, even longer.

The rabies vaccine is required by law in New York State where Bullet and I live. When Bullet was diagnosed with lymphoma, he had recently had an annual exam and vaccinations, including a three-year rabies vaccine. I didn't think that Bullet would outlive the vaccine.

Bullet's rabies vaccine expired in October of 2002. When the New York dog license renewal form arrived that year, it requested proof of current rabies vaccination. Our veterinarian filled out a waiver, which I enclosed with the renewal form and a check. For the past two years, the waiver has been accepted and Bullet's license to be a dog has been renewed without question.

REQUESTING A VACCINE WAIVER

‣ Dog's name, date of birth, breed, color and sex
‣ Owner's name and address
‣ According to the manufacturer's literature about the rabies vaccine, the product can be safely administered to healthy animals.
‣ The dog named above has been diagnosed with [type of cancer] and therefore administration of the vaccine to this animal could be dangerous to his health.
‣ The dog named above is free from infectious, contagious and/or communicable disease and is in good condition.
‣ According to the owner, there has been no known exposure to rabies or other communicable diseases within [ ] months and the dog

has not bitten anyone within the last 10 days.
- The county of residence is not under a rabies quarantine.
- The form should be dated and signed by your veterinarian with his or her license number.

OTHER PREVENTIVES

Heartworm preventives and products that protect your dog from flea and tick bites may or may not be problematic for a dog with cancer. I apologize for not taking a stand. Some veterinarians and some owners claim that these products should not be used on a dog with cancer; others claim that they are perfectly safe. There are varying opinions on this subject among veterinarians and I have no strong belief in either position.

If you live in an area where heartworm disease, flea infestation or tick bites are not common, you may decide to go without preventive and chance it. Ask your veterinarian how many cases there have been in the past few years.

During the second half of the summer of 2000, after Bullet's diagnosis, I did not apply heartworm preventive or flea and tick repellent. In the summer of 2001, I feared I was pushing my luck and used Frontline® every three months and Interceptor® every month and a half (this was a compromise, since both products recommend more frequent application). In the summer of 2002, I didn't use either. I was afraid to use them and afraid not to. I was compromising—using the preventives every other year—and praying.

Bullet became very ill in November 2002 and I feared heartworm. He was coughing and gagging intermittently and I cursed myself for not having used preventive. As it turned out, the cause of the coughing was not heartworm, but heart failure.

For those who would rather avoid mainstream preventives, there are natural products that may provide protection. Nosodes, for example, may protect a dog against a particular disease. Nosodes formulated for canine heartworm disease may protect a dog from contracting the disease, or can be given as a remedy after a dog has heartworm disease. Nosodes are homeopathic remedies formulated from the disease itself, as are vaccines. Brewer's yeast (mixed with a dog's food) and a variety of natural sprays also help to keep fleas and/or ticks at bay.

Periodic titer tests are extremely important for those who forgo vaccines. If you opt not to use preventives, consider titer testing twice a year for any disease against which your dog hasn't been vaccinated.

VACCINES AND CANINE CANCER PATIENTS

by Dr. W. Jean Dodds

Although vaccines are necessary and generally safe and efficacious, they can be ineffective at best and harmful at worst to dogs in selected situations. A vaccine can overwhelm a healthy animal with a genetic predisposition for adverse response to viral challenge. Seemingly healthy dogs harboring latent viral infections may not be able to withstand the additional immunological challenge induced by modified live virus (MLV) vaccines.

Vaccination can overwhelm an immuno-compromised dog. With cancer, the situation is complex because the mere presence of cancer cells can suppress immune function. Cancer-producing viral agents and other chemical carcinogens add to this immune onslaught, leaving the dog at high risk for an adverse reaction to vaccine.

After vaccination with MLV vaccine, a period of viremia begins on the 3rd to 14th day and continues for 2 to 4 weeks. During this period, the immune system activates the dog's cell-mediated response pathways which, in turn, may suppress immune surveillance mechanisms and either permit cancer cell regrowth or aggravate existing cancers.

Currently, about 15 percent of human tumors are known to be caused or enhanced by virus. Viruses also cause a number of tumors in animals and there is no doubt that the number of viruses found to do so will increase as techniques to isolate them improve.

The rising incidence of leukemia and lymphomas in an increasing number of dog breeds is a case in point. T-cell leukemias are associated with retroviral infections. Retroviral infections have also been associated with the production of autoimmunity and immunodeficiency diseases.

Similarly, there has been an increase in the incidence of hemangiosarcomas (malignant tumors of the blood vessel lining cells), primarily in the spleen but also in the heart, liver and skin. They occur most often in middle age or older dogs of medium to large breeds.

The German Shepherd dog is the breed at highest risk for hemangiosarcoma, but other breeds (including the Golden Retriever, Old English Sheepdog, Irish Setter and Vizsla) have shown a significantly increased incidence, especially in certain families. Thus, genetic and environmental influences predispose individual animals to immune dysfunction, which can result in adverse reactions when exposed to vaccines, certain drugs and toxins.

It's tempting to speculate that environmental factors that promote immune suppression or immune dysregulation, including vaccines, can lead to the failure of the immune surveillance mechanisms that protect the body against cancer-causing agents. Also, the cumulative effect of a lifetime of vaccinations may have consequences for a dog in later life, including an increased susceptibility to chronic debilitating diseases.

W. Jean Dodds, DVM, is president of Hemopet, a nonprofit animal blood bank and greyhound rescue/adoption program that also focuses on clinical research in diagnostic veterinary medicine through its Hemolife division. Dr. Dodds speaks to veterinary and kennel club groups throughout North America and overseas on vaccination issues, autoimmunity (hematology, immunology, thyroid and endocrine disorders) and nutrition.

Heartworm disease can be fatal but if detected early, it often can be cured. Lyme disease can be squashed by a course of antibiotics—again, early detection results in the best prognosis. In some cases, the disease persists and can cause long term lameness and/or neurologic symptoms.

BE PREPARED

In my experience, pets become ill most often on a Sunday or late at night. Stock a first-aid kit with items that you might need, including:

▸ L-Glutamine, pepcid AC and elderberry syrup for nausea
▸ PeptoBismol for diarrhea
▸ Metronidozole for mucousy diarrhea (Rx)

▸ A pain medication (This could be an over the counter medication such as an NSAID or a prescription drug. Ask your veterinarian to make a recommendation.
▸ Rescue Remedy, a homeopathic Bach Flower Essence remedy for stress.

Always be prepared for a real emergency. Check your local telephone book to find out where the nearest 24-hour emergency veterinary clinic is.

If you have a cell phone, program the clinic's telephone number into its memory. If you're not familiar with the location of the clinic, write or print out directions and keep this in your car or wallet. You might also take a ride there just to be sure that in an emergency situation, you will know how to get there quickly.

References

1   *Dr. Pitcairn's Complete Guide to Natural Health for Dogs & Cats*, by Richard H. Pitcairn, DVM, PhD. St. Martin's Press, 1995, p. 247.

THE MAGIC BULLET

~ PART TWO

Throughout Bullet's 75-week chemotherapy protocol, I saw him as a cancer-dog. My thoughts about him were tinged by the inevitability that at some time—perhaps today or perhaps a year from today—his remission would lapse; he would have chemotherapy side effects; he would slip into cancer cachexia. After years of remission, thoughts of cancer no longer echoed in my mind when I looked at or thought of Bullet.

My boy began the VELCAP-L chemotherapy protocol on July 18, 2000 and completed it in March 2002. He was 9½ going into chemotherapy, 11 coming out and getting into his senior years. I was truly offended the first time Dr. Hoskins referred to Bully as a "geriatric dog." How dare he? Ironically, I now refer to Bullet as a geriatric dog with pride.

During the six months after the end of Bullet's chemotherapy, I saw continual improvement in his health. His posture, his coat quality, eating habits and energy level—even his facial expressions—were once again that of a healthy dog. It took approximately six months for Bullet to recover fully from chemotherapy, but he did once again become strong, healthy and energetic, playful and happy.

Bullet was again able to go for long hikes and, as he regained his willful, playful husky personality, we fell back into our routine of arguing over which trail to hike, which toy to toss around, when to get into or out of the car and other very important decisions. He was able to spend long weekends with his furry friends running on the beach in Cape Cod.

In November 2002, Bullet developed a cough that sounded very much like a cat with fur balls: *"cough, cough, cough, gag."* Being an experienced cat caretaker, I was so sure of my "diagnosis" that I gave Bullet a hairball remedy marketed for felines for two days. The coughing persisted and so off to Dr. Hoskins we went.

Diagnostic tests revealed that Bullet's lungs were filled with fluid because his heart wasn't pumping properly. EKG and ultrasound testing rendered diagnoses of dilated cardiomyopathy and atrial fibrillation. My initial response was that this was an extremely unfair turn of events. Wasn't it enough that he had endured cancer and chemotherapy? Then, of course, I remembered that this didn't earn him immortality.

If we could get the fluid out of Bullet's lungs and control his heart conditions with medicine, he could survive another six months or a year. The medications did clear his lungs of fluid—the same medicines that are given to humans with these diagnoses, just as the chemotherapy agents used to fight canine cancer are the same as those that treat human cancer.

Bullet had a second cardiac event in April 2003, with the same coughing symptoms as the first. After a consultation with a board certified veterinary cardiologist at the Cornell University College of Veterinary Medicine, Dr. Hoskins adjusted the dosages of Bullet's medications and the fluid once again cleared from his lungs.

In April 2003, Bullet and I participated in the "Dogswalk Against Cancer," an event sponsored by the American Cancer Society to raise funds for cancer research. $2,000 of the money raised at this event was granted to the Cornell University College of Veterinary Medicine for the treatment of animals with cancer. Bullet completed the mile-and-a-half walk in good form and befriended a Girl Scout troop along the way (see photograph, page 75).

In August 2003, while visiting our friends in Cape Cod, Bullet's neck and throat region became so full that he had no neck to speak of. The lymph nodes were not enlarged but the entire area felt "mushy." The next morning, Bullet was lying on his side with no interest in getting up. His belly had become distended and hard overnight and I knew he was in serious trouble.

We were guests at the Bed and Breakfast of Margot and Dick Basile, dear friends and dog lovers par excellence. Complete and proper dog care is a top (if not *the* top) priority in the Basile household. Their veterinarian made a house call to examine Bullet and directed me to get him to a clinic post haste—one with an ultrasound unit. Naturally, this happened on a Saturday afternoon when most clinics are closed.

There ensued a frenzy of phone calls to local veterinary clinics, to Dr. Porzio, Dr. Hoskins and old acquaintances at Tufts Veterinary School of Veterinary Medicine because it was only a two-hour drive away.

My friend, her two dogs and Bullet and I packed the car in minutes and piled in. After a two-hour drive, Bullet stayed overnight at the Foster Small Animal Hospital, the 24-hour emergency clinic at Tufts University School of Veterinary Medicine in North Grafton, MA. With a nitroglycerine patch on his ear, an injection of lasix and constant monitoring, his condition improved marginally overnight. In the morning, I checked him out to move him to an emergency clinic near home.

After another two-hour white-knuckle car ride with two humans and three dogs, we arrived at the 24-hour emergency animal hospital in Bedford, NY. In response to a "heads up" call by cell phone ten minutes before our arrival, two staff workers were waiting for us in the parking lot with a gurney, ready to transport Bullet from my car into the hospital.

There were diagnostic tests and revisions in Bullet's cardiac medications, and he recovered once again but was not his old spunky self. Dr. Porzio suggested I research a cardiac medication for dogs not yet approved for use in the U.S. After finding a pharmacist willing to export the drug from Great Britain to Dr. Hoskins, I procured FDA permission to import the drug.

Via the Internet, I was able to correspond with several people whose dogs had been given this medication and they all claimed that their dogs survived several years with good quality of life because of this drug. I can now concur—Bullet's energy level and quality of life improved greatly. He regained his spunk and his "growly bear" personality.

On March 15, 2004, Bullet turned 13 years old. At the 2004 Dogswalk Against Cancer, he was selected as King of the Dogswalk. Coincidentally, his Queens were Diamond Dreamer and Suzi, cancer-dogs whose caretakers I met online at one of the Pet Cancer Support Groups.

In May, I discovered a tumor on Bullet's side. I immediately stopped feeding him oatmeal and reinstated his cancer supplements. A needle biopsy indicated that the tumor was a spindle cell tumor and was most probably malignant. Removal of the tumor with wide margins was the recommendation. "How would you feel," I asked Dr. Hoskins, "about operating on a 13-year-old Husky with lymphoma and heart disease?"

The tumor was removed with wide margins. As advised by Dr. Ruslander, the surgery was performed by a board certified surgeon with the assistance of Dr. Hoskins. Bullet came through the surgery in reasonably good shape and as this book goes to print, he is recuperating nicely.

Bullet's home-care regimen has become fairly complicated what with the cardiac medications and supplements plus cancer medications and supplements, not to mention diapering when he's indoors. But, as with everything, a routine has developed and it's become less complicated than it sounds. Fortunately—or perhaps I should say unfortunately—we've had lots of practice.

Bullet has now maintained one long remission from lymphoma for nearly four years and has survived heart disease for more than eighteen months with four episodes of congestive heart failure. I missed the first 18 months of Bullet's life and I'm very grateful that I have been given the opportunity to keep him by my side during his twilight years. I'm grateful to Bullet's cancer team and cardiac team and to all of the veterinarians who have treated Bullet with such great care and expertise. I'm grateful to our wonderful friends, Bullet's Aunts and Uncles, who have cared for him when I could not and who have been supportive to us both through thick and thin.

This is the story of a very special dog, "the love of my life; the dog of my dreams." It's the story of a shelter dog who was once named Max but came to be known as Bullet. Who earned the titles of Bully, Bullet Growly Bear and King Bully and who will now be known always as The Magic Bullet.

RESOURCES

RECOMMENDED READING

Animals as Guides for the Soul, by Susan Chernak McElroy. The Ballentine Publishing Group, 1998.

Beating Cancer with Nutrition, by Patrick Quillin, PhD, RD, CNS with Noreen Quillin. Nutrition Times Press, Inc., 2001.

Complete Guide to Natural Health for Dogs & Cats, by Richard H. Pitcairn, DVM, PhD, and Susan Hubble Pitcairn. St. Martin's Press, 1995.

Food Pets Die For: Shocking Facts about Pet Food, by Ann. N. Martin. New Sage Press, 2003.

Holistic Guide for a Healthy Dog, by Wendy Volhard and Kerry Brown, DVM. Howell Book House, 2000.

Home Safe Home: Protecting Yourself and Your Family from Everyday Toxics and Harmful Household Products in the Home, by Debra Dadd-Redalia and Debra Lynn Dadd. J. P. Tarcher, 1997.

Kindred Spirits: How the Remarkable Bond Between Humans and Animals Can Change the Way We Live, by Allen M. Schoen, M.S. D.V.M. Broadway, 2001.

Manual of Natural Veterinary Medicine: Science and Tradition, by Susan G. Wynn, DVM and Steve Marsden. Mosby, 2002.

Natural Health Bible for Dogs & Cats, by Shawn Messonnier, DVM. Prima Publishing, 2001.

Natural Nutrition for Dogs and Cats, by Kymythy R. Schulze, CCN, AHI. Hay House, Inc., 1998.

Pets Living With Cancer, by Robin Downing, DVM. AAHA Press, 2000.

Small Animal Clinical Oncology, editors Stephen J. Withrow, DVM, diplomate ACVIM (oncology) and E. Gregory MacEwen, VMD, diplomate ACVIM (oncology and internal medicine). W.B. Saunders Company, 2001.

Small Animal Internal Medicine, by Richard W. Nelson, G. Guillermo Couto etc. al. Mosby, Inc., 1999.

Survive Your Cancer: The Essential Who, What, Where, When & How Guide for Cancer Patients & Their Families, by Barbara Brandon. Survivor's Wisdom, 2003.

The Complete Herbal Handbook for the Dog and Cat, by Juliette De Bairacli Levy. Faber & Faber, 1991.

The Essential Guide to Natural Pet Care: Cancer, by Cal Orey. BowTie Press, 1998.

The Illustrated Veterinary Guide, Second Edition, by Chris C. Pinney, DVM. McGraw-Hill, 2000.

The Nature of Animal Healing: The Definitive Holistic Medicine Guide to Caring for Your Dog and Cat, by Marty Goldstein, DVM. Ballantine Books, 2000.

The Naturally Clean Home: 101 Safe and Easy Herbal Formulas for Non-Toxic Cleansers, by Karyn Siegel-Maier. Workman Publishing Company, 1999.

The Rainbow Bridge, by Paul C. Dahm. Running Tide Press, 1997.

The Veterinarian's Guide to Natural Remedies for Dogs, by Martin Zucker. Three Rivers Press, 1999.

Why is Cancer Killing Our Pets?, by Deborah Straw. Healing Arts Press, 2000.

GENERAL INFORMATION

American College of Veterinary Internal Medicine
Phone: (800) 245-9081
Web site: [www.acvim.org]

Animal Cancer Institute
Web site: [www.animalcancerinstitute.com]

Animal Poison Control Center
Phone: (888) 426-4435
Web site: [www.apcc.aspca.org]

Morris Animal Foundation
Phone: (800) 243-2345
Website: [www.morrisanimalfoundation.org]

The Perseus Foundation
Web site: [www.perseusfoundation.org]

Veterinary Cancer Society
Phone: (619) 474-8929
Web site: [www.vetcancersociety.org]

PRODUCTS

Home Harvest Garden Supply, Inc.
Phone: (800) 348-4769
Website: [http://homeharvest.com]

Peaceful Valley Farm Supply
Phone: (888) 784-1722
Web site: [www.groworganic.com]

Poly MVA® (AMARC Enterprises, Inc.)
Phone: (800) 960-6760
Web site: [www.polymva.com]

Hug-a-Dog Harness from D3Pet Productions
Phone (800) 444-9475
Web site: [www.hug-a-dog.com]

Safety Seat Support Harness™
Four Paws® Products Ltd.
Phone: (631) 434-1100
Web site: [www.fourpaws.com]

3-in-1 Vest Harness™ Dog Safety Restraint
RC Pet Products
Phone: (604) 272-5253
Web site: [www.vetbuy.com]

THE MAGIC BULLET FUND

If you're reading this, you've already made your first contribution!

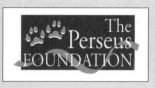

A portion of the proceeds generated from sales of the book, *Help Your Dog Fight Cancer* will be donated to a charitable organization to benefit dogs with cancer.

The paragraph you see above has been sitting on this page for a long time, awaiting definition. Surely, I thought, such an organization exists. Surely, I'll find it before completing the book. As *Help Your Dog Fight Cancer* neared completion, I had not found it.

During a last-minute search, I contacted The Perseus Foundation and reached its president, Tom Nelson. I told Tom about this book, about Bullet and about my search for an organization that provides financial assistance to caretakers of dogs with cancer.

Tom Nelson and The Perseus Foundation have made my dream come true. It's not my dream alone—it's the dream of thousands of cancer-dog caretakers who are struggling to accept the harsh reality that they are unable to provide cancer treatment for their adoring and adored canine friends.

The Magic Bullet Fund has been established in honor of Bullet and under the umbrella of The Perseus Foundation. Tom wasted no time getting the fund off to a running start. Veterinary oncologists across the country have been enlisted to provide cancer treatment on behalf of The Magic Bullet Fund. A top distributor of veterinary pharmaceuticals has graciously agreed to donate chemotherapy agents to be administered to dogs receiving treatment through the Fund.

The Magic Bullet Fund provides all caretakers of dogs with cancer with the possibility of pursuing treatment for their beloved pets. When you purchased this book, you made your first contribution to the Fund.

Please give again!
Give to help more dogs survive cancer.

Send a check payable to" The Magic Bullet Fund"
Send to: The Perseus Foundation
1432 120th Street, New Richmond, WI 54017

Donate Online:
[www.perseusfoundation.org/TheMagicBulletFund]

Request Assistance:
[www.perseusfoundation.org/TheMagicBulletFund]
or call (715) 246-2454.

Many thanks from me, Bullet and all of the dogs who will benefit from your generosity.